ABC OF ASTHMA

Fifth Edition

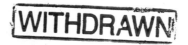

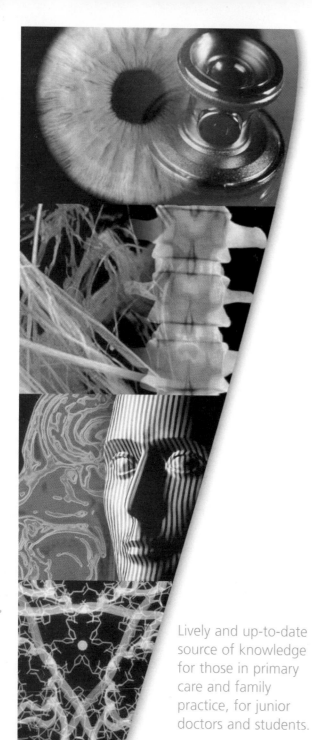
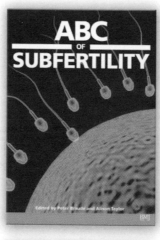
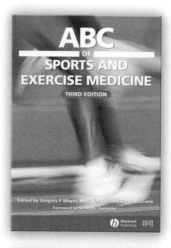
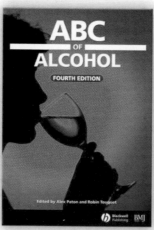
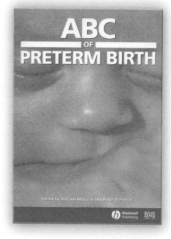
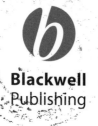
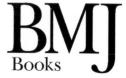

ABC OF ASTHMA

Fifth Edition

JOHN REES
Senior lecturer and consultant physician,
Guy's, King's and St Thomas' School of Medicine, London

DIPAK KANABAR
Consultant paediatrician,
Guy's, King's and St Thomas' School of Medicine, London

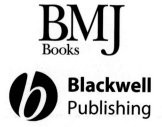

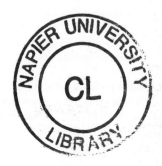

Blackwell Publishing Inc., 350 Main Street, Malden, Massachusetts 02148-5020, USA
Blackwell Publishing Ltd, 9600 Garsington Road, Oxford OX4 2DQ, UK
Blackwell Publishing Asia Pty Ltd, 550 Swanston Street, Carlton, Victoria 3053, Australia

First published 1984
Second edition 1989
Third edition 1995
Fourth edition 2000
Fifth edition 2006

Library of Congress Cataloging-in-Publication Data

Rees, John, 1949–
        ABC of asthma/John Rees, Dipak Kanabar. — 5th ed.
            p.   ;   cm.
        Includes bibliographical references and index.
        ISBN-13: 978-0-7279-1860-4 (alk. paper)
        ISBN-10: 0-7279-1860-5 (alk. paper)
        1. Asthma.   I. Kanabar, Dipak.   II. Title.
        [DNLM: 1. Asthma.   WF 553 R328a 2005]
    RC591.R43 2005
    616.2'38—dc22

                                                                            2005020704

ISBN-13: 978 0 7279 1860 4
ISBN-10: 0 7279 1860 5

A catalogue record for this book is available from the British Library

The cover shows allergens in the trachea. With permission from Eddy Gray/Science Photo Library

Set in 9/11 pt New Baskerville by Newgen Imaging Systems (P) Ltd, Chennai, India
Printed and bound in India by Replika Press Pvt. Ltd, Harayana

Commissioning Editor: Eleanor Lines
Technical Editor: Barbara Squire
Development Editors: Sally Carter, Nick Morgan
Production Controller: Debbie Wyer

For further information on Blackwell Publishing, visit our website:
http://www.blackwellpublishing.com

The publisher's policy is to use permanent paper from mills that operate a sustainable forestry policy,
and which has been manufactured from pulp processed using acid-free and elementary chlorine-free
practices. Furthermore, the publisher ensures that the text paper and cover board used have met
acceptable environmental accreditation standards.

Contents

ASTHMA IN ADULTS – John Rees

1 Definition and pathology

Asthma is a common condition that has increased in prevalence throughout the world over the past 30 years. There is no precise universally agreed definition of asthma. The descriptive statements that exist include references to inflammation in the lungs, increased responsiveness of the airways, and reversibility of the airflow obstruction.

The clinical picture of asthma in young adults is recognisable and reproducible. The difficulties in precise diagnosis come in the very young, in older people, and in very mild asthma. Breathlessness from other causes, such as the increased tendency to obesity, may be confused with asthma.

The clinical characteristic of asthma is airflow obstruction that can be reversed over short periods of time or with treatment. This may be evident from provocation by specific stimuli or from the response to bronchodilator drugs. The airflow obstruction leads to the usual symptoms of shortness of breath. The underlying pathology is inflammatory change in the airway wall leading to irritability and responsiveness to various stimuli—and also to coughing, the other common symptom of asthma.

Asthma has commonly been defined on the basis of wide variations over short periods of time in resistance to airflow. Recent definitions have come to recognise the importance of the inflammatory change in the airways.

Low concentrations of non-specific stimuli—such as inhaled methacholine and histamine—produce airway narrowing. In general, the more severe the asthma the greater the inflammation and the more the airways react on challenge. Other stimuli—such as cold air, exercise, and hypotonic solutions—can also provoke this increased reactivity. In contrast, it is difficult to induce *significant* narrowing of the airways with many of these stimuli in healthy people. In some epidemiological studies increased airway responsiveness is used as part of the definition of asthma. Wheezing during the past 12 months is added to exclude those who have increased responsiveness but no symptoms.

In clinical practice in the UK airway responsiveness demonstrated in the laboratory is not often used in the diagnosis of asthma. The clinical equivalent of the increased responsiveness is development of symptoms in response to dust, smoke, cold air, and exercise; these should be sought in the history.

Labelling

In the past there was a tendency to use the term "wheezy bronchitis" in children rather than "asthma" in the belief that this would protect the parents from the label of asthma.

More recently there has been a greater inclination to label and treat mild wheezing or breathlessness as asthma. These diagnostic trends have been seen in studies of prevalence. Studies through the 1970s and 1980s showed increasing prevalence, emergency room attendance, admission, and even mortality, but recent studies suggest a levelling off or decline in these more severe markers and of self reported wheezing, though the prevalence of the use of label of asthma has remained high or continued to increase.

The International Consensus Report on the Diagnosis and Management of Asthma gives the following definition: "Asthma is a chronic inflammatory disorder of the airway in which many cells play a role, in particular mast cells, eosinophils, and T lymphocytes. In susceptible individuals this inflammation causes recurrent episodes of wheezing, breathlessness, chest tightness, and cough, particularly at night or in the early morning. These symptoms are usually associated with widespread but variable airflow limitation that is at least partly reversible either spontaneously or with treatment. The inflammation also causes an associated increase in airway responsiveness to a variety of stimuli."

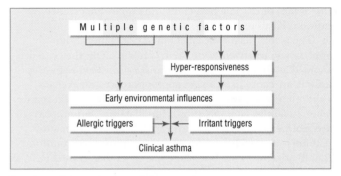

Genetics and the environment influence asthma

THE
PREFACE
TO THE
TREATISE
OF THE
ASTHMA

SINCE the Cure of the *Asthma* is observed by all Physicians, who have attempted the Eradicating that Chronical Distemper, to be very difficult, and frequently unsuccessful; I may thence infer, That either the true Nature of that Disease is not thoroughly understood by them, or they have not yet found out the Medicines by which the Cure may be effected.

It is my Design in this Treatise, to enquire more particularly into the Nature of this Disease; and, according to that Notion I can give of it, to propose those Methods and Medicines which appear to me most likely to effect its Cure, or, at least, to palliate it.

B

The preface to *The Treatise of the Asthma* by J Floyer, published in 1717

The relevance of early environment has been increasingly evident in epidemiological studies. A considerable degree of the future risk of asthma and course of disease seems to depend on factors before or shortly after birth.

Self reported wheezing in the past 12 months is used as the criterion for diagnosing asthma in many epidemiological studies. Wheezing is a very common symptom, affecting three quarters of participants at some time in a recent study of people followed up to the age of 26.

In most people with asthma, available treatments can suppress symptoms to allow normal activity without significant adverse effects. These are the goals of most asthma guidelines. Treatments, however, are not always delivered efficiently, and many people with milder asthma remain symptomatic. Only a few people have difficult to control asthma or troublesome side effects of treatment. In contrast, though we understand more about the onset and natural course of asthma, little practical advance has yet been made in its cure or prevention.

In infants under the age of 2 wheezing is common because of the small size of the airways. Many of these affected infants will not go on to wheeze later. In adults who smoke, asthma may be difficult to differentiate from narrowing of the airways that is part of chronic bronchitis and emphysema caused by previous cigarette smoking.

The actual diagnostic label would not matter if the appropriate treatment were used. Unfortunately, the evidence shows that children and adults who are diagnosed as having asthma are more likely to get appropriate treatment than children with the same symptoms who are given an alternative label. In adults, attempts at bronchodilatation and prophylaxis are more extensive in those who are labelled as asthmatic. Asthma is now such a common and well publicised condition that the diagnosis tends to cause less upset than it used to. With adequate explanation most patients and parents will accept it. The correct treatment can then be started. Persistent problems of cough and wheeze are likely to be much more worrying than the correct diagnosis and improvement in symptoms on treatment. The particular problems of the diagnosis of asthma in very young children are dealt with in chapter 12 (p.51).

Treating older patients

In older patients the most common dilemma is differentiation from chronic obstructive pulmonary disease (COPD). As both conditions are common, some patients will have both. A degree of increased airway responsiveness is found in COPD in relation to geometry from the narrower airways and the 20% change defining responsiveness. Bronchodilators can be used for both conditions, although the agent may vary (p.36). Inhaled corticosteroids are a mainstay early treatment of asthma, but in COPD they are reserved for more severe disease or frequent exacerbations. When there is doubt they should be used.

Pathology

Since the 1990s there has been more interest in and understanding of inflammation in the asthmatic airway. Inflammation in the airway wall involves oedema, infiltration with various cells, disruption and detachment of the epithelial layer, and hypertrophy of mucus glands. Changes occur in the subepithelial layer, with the laying down of forms of collagen and other extracellular matrix proteins.

This remodelling of the airway wall in response to persistent inflammation can resolve but may result in permanent fibrotic damage, possibly related to the irreversible airflow obstruction that may develop in poorly controlled asthma.

Differential diagnosis in adults

Chronic obstructive pulmonary disease
- May be difficult to differentiate from chronic asthma in older smokers
- The pathology differs, as does the degree of responsiveness to steroids

Large airway obstruction
- Caused by tumours, strictures, and foreign bodies; often misdiagnosed as asthma initially
- Differentiated by flow volume loop (see p.12)

Pulmonary oedema
- Once called "cardiac asthma"
- May mimic asthma, including the presence of wheezing and worsening at night

---

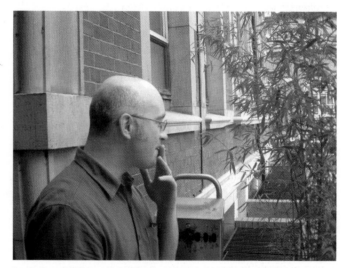

In smokers COPD may be difficult to distinguish from chronic asthma

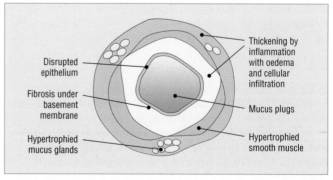

Inflammatory changes in the airway

There is evidence that symptoms in very early life are related to lifelong change in lung function. Early and prolonged intervention may be necessary to allow normal development of the airways and lungs and prevent permanent changes. In older children corticosteroids can suppress inflammation, but this returns, with associated hyper-responsiveness, when the drugs are stopped.

The inflammatory cells involved in asthma include eosinophils, mast cells, lymphocytes, and neutrophils. Dendritic cells, derived from monocytes, present antigen and induce proliferation in naive T cells and primed Th2 cells. Antigen cross links IgE to produce activation and degranulation of mast cells. T lymphocytes seem to have a controlling influence on the characteristic inflammation. Th2 lymphocytes that produce interleukin 4, 5, 9, and 13 are more common in the airway in asthma. Inflammatory cells are attracted to the airway by chemokines and then bind to adhesion molecules on the vessel endothelium. From there they migrate in to the local tissue.

In acute inflammatory conditions such as pneumonia the processes usually resolve. In asthma chronic inflammation can disrupt the normal repair process; growth factors are produced by inflammatory and tissue cells to produce a remodelling of the airway. There is proliferation of smooth muscle and blood vessels with fibrosis and thickening of the basement membrane. Thickened smooth muscle increases responsiveness and, together with fibrosis, reduces airway calibre. Some of these changes may be reversible, but others can lead to permanent damage and reduced reversibility in chronic asthma.

Clinical evidence

Early evidence on the changes in the airway wall came from a few studies of postmortem material. The understanding advanced with the use of bronchial biopsies taken at bronchoscopy. These studies showed that, even in remission, there is persistent inflammation in the airway wall.

Cells from the alveoli and small airways obtained by alveolar lavage can give another measure of airway inflammation. However, this cannot be repeated regularly and is not practical as a monitor in clinical practice. Induced sputum, produced in response to breathing hypertonic saline, is an alternative more acceptable method.

All these techniques sample different areas and cell populations and by themselves may induce changes that affect repeated studies. They have, however, provided valuable information on cellular and mediator changes and the effects of treatment or airway challenge.

A simpler method entails analysis of expired air. This has been used to measure exhaled nitric oxide produced by nitric oxide synthase, which is increased in the inflamed asthmatic airway. Other possibilities are measurement of pH of the expired breath condensate, carbon monoxide as a sign of oxidative stress, or products of arachidonic acid metabolism such as 8-isoprostane. These methods hold promise for simpler methods of measuring airway inflammation but are not routinely used.

Mucus plugging

In severe asthma, there is mucus plugging within the lumen and loss of parts of the surface epithelium. Extensive mucus plugging is the striking finding in the lungs of patients who die of an acute exacerbation of asthma.

Asthma as a general condition

It has been suggested that asthma is a generalised abnormality of the inflammatory or immune cells and that the lungs are just the site where the symptoms show. This does not explain the

> Some of the inflammatory changes in the airway wall can be reduced or prevented by suitable therapy. The point at which the changes become irreversible is uncertain

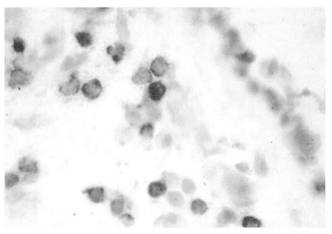

CD3 positive lymphocytes in mucosa (courtesy of Chris Corrigan)

> A key question is whether early, effective anti-inflammatory treatment can prevent inflammatory changes to the airway wall producing irreversible change

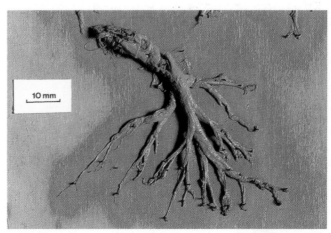

10 mm

Extensive airway plugs and casts of airways can occur in severe asthma

finding that lungs from a donor with mild asthma transplanted into a patient without asthma produced problems with obstruction of airflow, while normal lungs transplanted into a patient with asthma were free from problems. The link to the nasal mucosa, however, has been recognised more widely. The same trigger factors may affect both areas of the respiratory tract. A combined approach to treatment may be helpful in control of each area.

Types of asthma

Most asthma develops during childhood and usually varies considerably with time and treatment. Young patients usually have identifiable triggers that provoke wheezing, though there is seldom one single extrinsic cause for all their attacks. This "extrinsic" asthma is often associated with other features of atopy such as rhinitis and eczema. When asthma starts in adult life the airflow obstruction is often more persistent and many exacerbations have no obvious stimuli other than respiratory tract infections. This pattern is often called "intrinsic" asthma. Immediate skin prick tests are less likely to yield positive results because of a lack of involvement of allergens or a loss of skin test positivity with age.

Other categories

There are many patients who do not fit into these broad groups or who overlap the two types. There are other important types of asthma, including presentation with just a cough and asthma related to occupational exposure.

Presentation with a cough is particularly common in children. Even in adults it should be considered as the cause of chronic unexplained cough. In some series of such cases, asthma, or a combination of rhinitis and asthma, explained the cough in about half the patients who had been troubled by a cough with no obvious cause for more than two months.

Churg-Strauss syndrome is a rare systemic vasculitis associated with asthma. The asthma is usually severe and often precedes other elements of the condition. The diagnostic criteria include asthma, blood and tissue eosinophilia, and vasculitis. Treatment is with corticosteroids and other immunosuppressants, as well as appropriate treatment for the asthma, which may be difficult to control.

Types of asthma

Childhood onset
- Most asthma starts in childhood, usually in atopic children
- Tends to have considerable variability and identifiable precipitants

Adult onset
- Often a relapse of earlier asthma, but may have initial onset at any age
- Often more persistent with fewer obvious precipitants except infection

Nocturnal
- Common in all types of asthma
- Related to poor overall control and increased reactivity

Occupational
- Underdiagnosed
- Needs expert evaluation

Cough variant
- Cough is a common symptom and may precede airflow obstruction

Exercise induced
- Common precipitant
- May be the only significant precipitant in children

Brittle
- Two types:
  Chaotic uncontrolled asthma with variable peak flow
  Sudden severe deteriorations from a stable baseline

Aspirin sensitive
- May be associated with later onset and nasal polyps
- Only 2-3% have a history of asthma but formal tests identify asthma in 10-20%

Churg-Strauss syndrome
- An uncommon diffuse vasculitis characterised by severe persistent asthma
- Initial clue may be high eosinophilia ($>1500/\mu l$) or vasculitic involvement of another organ

---

Further reading

- Chronic obstructive pulmonary disease. National clinical guideline on management of chronic obstructive pulmonary disease in adults in primary and secondary care. *Thorax* 2004;59(suppl 1):1-232.
- International Consensus Report on the Diagnosis and Management of Asthma. *Clin Exper Allergy* 1992; suppl 1:1-72.
- Sears MR, Greene JM, Willan AR, Wiecek EM, Taylor DR, Flannery EM, et al. A longitudinal, population-based cohort study of childhood asthma followed to adulthood. *N Engl J Med* 2003;349:1414-22.

2 Prevalence

Genetics

There have been considerable advances recently in understanding the genetics of asthma. A familial link has been recognised for some time together with an association with allergic rhinitis and allergic eczema. The familial link with atopic disorders is strongest in childhood asthma and with the link to maternal atopy. Earlier investigations were helped by studies of isolated communities—such as in Tristan da Cunha, where the high prevalence of asthma can be traced to three women among the original settlers.

Genetic studies

Early studies of genetic links within families with more than one member with asthma suggested a strong link to certain genetic regions of interest, particularly 5q and 11q. Further studies in different populations did not replicate all the early findings, and it became evident that, as in other common conditions, the genetic links were not simple. Several issues have been identified, and there seem to be differences in the links between ethnic groups. Susceptibility seems to be determined by several genes that have an effect in different aspects of asthma. There has been steady progress moving from areas of broad linkage to candidate asthma genes. Again, findings have not always been replicated in different populations. Genes have been identified that are linked to the Th2 cytokine signalling pathway, Th2 cell differentiation, airway remodelling, innate and adaptive immune responses, and IgE levels. Most of the work relates to the presence of asthma. Further work is investigating different asthma phenotypes and the natural course and severity of asthma, and interaction with environmental influences.

Future investigations

Future investigations in the genetics of asthma may teach us more about susceptibility and progression in asthma. Genetic influences may also underlie different responses to treatment and raise the promise of matching treatment to a patient's individual response and the production of new forms of therapy aimed at influencing specific genes and their products.

Early environment

Genetic susceptibility alone does not account for the development or persistence of asthma. Genetic susceptibility is linked to environmental exposure. Early environmental influences before and soon after birth may be particularly important. The type and extent of exposure to allergens and infections may influence the development of the immune process and the likelihood of the development of asthma.

The hygiene hypothesis links to this balance of the parts of the immune system. It was noted that asthma was less likely to develop in children with older siblings. The hypothesis is that processes such as earlier exposure to infections from older siblings and commensal gut bacteria may help the maturation of the immune system and the switch to a Th1 lymphocyte phenotype rather than the Th2 phenotype. The Th1 cellular immune responses are related to protection against many infections while Th2 responses favour atopy. This was supported by evidence that asthma and allergies are less common in children brought up on farms and in close contact with animals.

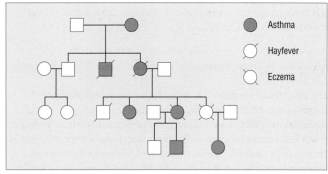

Family tree of an atopic family

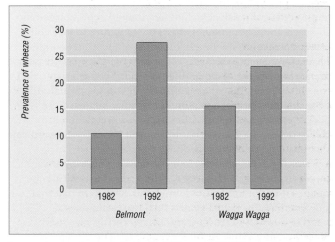

Increase in prevalence of wheeze in children aged 8-10 in two towns in New South Wales between 1982 and 1992. There was a pronounced increase in counts of house dust mite in domestic dust over the same period (Peat JK et al, *BMJ* 1994;308:1591-6)

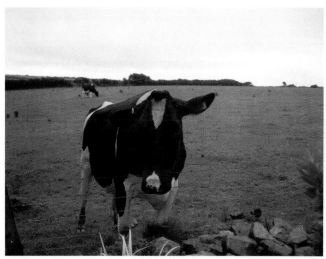

Early exposure to animals seems to reduce the risk of subsequent asthma

The hypothesis has been extended to suggest that, as well as immune maturation in infancy, the degree of competence of the immune system achieved at birth may be important. The influences on this are poorly understood but might be related to the prenatal cytokine environment.

Genetic factors and clinical course

Atopic people are at risk of asthma and rhinitis. They can be identified by immediate positive results from skin prick tests to common allergens

The development of asthma depends on environmental factors acting with a genetic predisposition. The movement of racial groups with a low prevalence of asthma from an isolated rural environment to an urban area increases the prevalence in that group, possibly because of their increased exposure to allergens such as house dust mites and fungal spores or to infectious agents, pollution, and dietary changes.

Family history—The chance of a person developing asthma by the age of 50 is 10 times higher if there is a first degree relative with asthma. The risk is greater the more severe the relative's asthma. It has been suggested that breast feeding could reduce the risk of a child developing atopic conditions such as asthma because it restricts the exposure to ingested foreign protein in the first few months of life. Conflicting results have been published, and it may require considerable dietary restriction by the mother to avoid passing antigen on to the child during this vulnerable period. Overall, though infant wheezing may be less common in breastfed infants, there is no good evidence to show that asthma is less prevalent. Nevertheless, the many other benefits of breast feeding indicate that it should be encouraged.

Smoking in pregnancy—Maternal smoking in pregnancy increases the risk of childhood asthma; exposure during the first few years of life is also detrimental. Studies of paternal smoking have produced similar but less certain trends.

Weight control—Obesity is associated with an increased likelihood of asthma. Regular exercise to maintain fitness and control weight is sensible advice for people with asthma.

Diagnostic criteria in epidemiological studies

For epidemiological purposes, a common set of criteria is the presence of symptoms in the previous 12 months and evidence of increased bronchial responsiveness. Phase 1 of the international study of asthma and allergies in childhood (ISAAC) looked at prevalence of symptoms in 13-14 year olds in 155 centres worldwide. Prevalence rates differed over 20-fold, and ISAAC phase 2 will explore these differences. The Odense study in children found 27% with current symptoms of asthma but only 10% were diagnosed as asthmatic. Different diagnostic tests, such as methacholine responsiveness, peak flow monitoring, and exercise testing, did not correlate well with each other. Each test was reasonably specific, but individual sensitivities were low. The combination of peak flow monitoring at home and methacholine responsiveness produced the best results.

Prevalence figures

The reported prevalence depends on the definition of asthma being used and the age and type of the studied population. Regional variations exist, particularly in developing countries, where rates in urban areas are higher than in poor rural

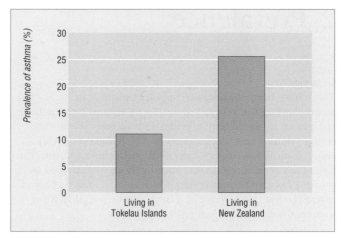

Prevalence of asthma in Tokelauan children aged 0–14 still in the Tokelau Islands or resettled to New Zealand. Asthma, rhinitis, and eczema were all more prevalent in islanders who had been settled in New Zealand after a hurricane. Environmental factors have an effect as well as genetic predisposition (Waite DA et al, *Clin All* 1980;10:71-5)

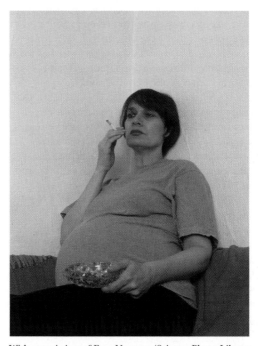

With permission of Faye Norman/Science Photo Library

The results of the Odense study confirm that no single physiological test is perfect and that different tests may detect different clinical aspects of asthma. A positive result on either test combined with a typical history would confirm the diagnosis of asthma

districts. For clinically *significant* asthma many countries have broad prevalence rates of around 5% in adults and 10% in children, but definitions based on hyper-responsiveness or wheeze in the past 12 months produce rates of around 30% in children.

In the past the label of asthma was possibly used more readily in social classes I and II, but more recent figure for young adults across Europe indicate a higher prevalence in lower socioeconomic groups, regardless of atopy.

Most studies using equivalent diagnostic criteria across the 1970s to 1990s showed that the prevalence of asthma was increasing. More recent studies show that this increase has reached a plateau or even reversed in developed countries. A recent study showed a decline from 29% to 24% in the symptom of wheeze in the previous year in Australian primary school children. ISAAC showed a similar decrease from 34% to 28% for 12-14 year olds between 1995 and 2002. Interestingly, the label of asthma, especially mild asthma, was being used more over this time

During the past 10 years admissions to hospital for asthma and emergency room attendances have declined, especially in children. This may be linked to better control through appropriate treatment. The pattern in developed countries suggests that prevalence peaked around 1990. While there has been an increasing tendency to use the label of asthma, the true prevalence and the frequency of more serious asthma is showing signs of a reduction.

The sex ratio in children aged around 7 shows that one and a half times to twice as many boys are affected as girls, but as teenagers boys do better than girls, and by the time they reach adulthood the sex incidence has become about equal.

Changes in prevalence

Several explanations were suggested for the increase in prevalence. The strong genetic element has not changed so any true increase, other than in changes in detection or diagnosis, must come from environmental factors. No single explanation is likely as the possible factors do not apply equally to all the populations experiencing the change in prevalence.

Change in the indoor environment—The advent of centrally heated homes with warm bedrooms, high humidity, and soft furnishings probably increases exposure to house dust mite. This may be part of the explanation but does not fit with changes in developing countries.

Smoking—Maternal smoking during pregnancy and infancy is associated with an increased prevalence of asthma in childhood. The increase in smoking among young women in recent years may play some part in the increase in prevalence. Smoking by people with asthma increases its persistence.

Family size—The reduction in family size, with the increased risk in first born children, plays a small part.

Pollution—Symptoms of asthma are made worse by atmospheric pollutions such as nitrogen sulphur dioxide and small particulate matter. However, outdoor environmental pollution levels do not correlate with changes in prevalence. Indoor pollution from oxides of nitrogen, organic compounds, and fungal spores may be more important.

Diet—Some studies have shown relations between diet and asthma related to higher salt intake, low selenium, or reduced vitamin C, vitamin E, or certain polysaturated fats. The effects of dietary intervention, however, have not supported or refuted this as a major contribution.

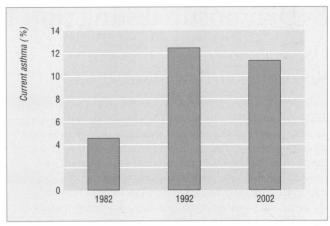

Prevalence of asthma in Australian children aged 8-11 has shown that the prevalence has reached a plateau (adapted from Toelle BG, et al. Prevalence of asthma and allergy in schoolchildren in Belmont, Australia: three cross sectional surveys over 20 years. *BMJ* 2004;328:386-7)

Possible explanation for changes in prevalence of asthma

- Indoor environment
- Smoking
- Family size
- Pollution
- Diet

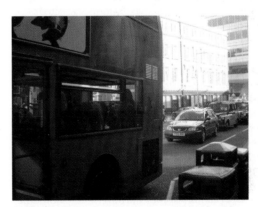

Outdoor pollution increase symptoms in people with asthma

Further reading

- Anderson HR, Ruggles R, Strachan DP, Austin JB, Burr M, Jeffs D, et al. Trends in prevalence of symptoms of asthma, hay fever, and eczema in 12-14 year olds in the British Isles, 1995-2002: questionnaire survey. *BMJ* 2004;328:1052-3.
- Basagana X, Sunyer J, Kogevinas M, Zock JP, Duan-Tauleria E, Jarvis D, et al. Socio-economic status and asthma prevalence in young adults: the European community health survey. *Am J Epidemiol* 2004;160:178-88.
- Peat JK, van den Berg RH, Green WF, Mellis CM, Leeder SR, Woolcock AJ. Changing prevalence of asthma in Australian children. *BMJ* 1994;308:1591-6.
- Siersted HC, Mostgaard G, Hyldebrandt N, Hansen HS, Boldsen J, Oxho JH. Interrelationships between diagnosed asthma, asthma-like symptoms, and abnormal airway behaviour in adolescence: the Odense school child study. *Thorax* 1996;51:503-9.
- Toelle BG, Ng K, Belousova E, Salome CM, Peat JK, Marks GB. Prevalence of asthma and allergy in schoolchildren in Belmont, Australia: three cross sectional surveys over 20 years. *BMJ* 2004;328:386-7.
- Wills-Karp M, Ewart SL. Time to draw breath: asthma susceptibility genes are identified. *Nature Review Genetics* 2004;5:376-87.

3 Diagnostic testing and monitoring

Recording airflow obstruction

Mini peak flow meters provide a simple method of measuring airflow obstruction. The measurements add an objective element to subjective feelings of shortness of breath. Several types are available. The traditional Wright peak flow meters have errors that vary over the range of measurement. As patients use the same peak flow meter over time they can build up a pattern of their asthma, which can be important in changing their treatment and planning management. In September 2004 meters became available that give accurate readings over the full range. These compare accurately with peak flow from other sources such as spirometry. It is important to explain this change clearly to patients and to adjust their management plans.

Particular encouragement to record peak flow should be given to:

- Poor perceivers, in whom symptoms do not reflect changes in objective measured obstruction
- Patients with a history of sudden exacerbations
- Patients with poor asthma control
- Times of adjustment in therapy, either up or down
- Situations where a link to a precipitating factor is suspected
- Periodic recordings in stable asthma to establish usual levels and confirm reliability of symptoms

---

Use of diary cards

Although acute attacks of asthma occasionally have a sudden catastrophic onset, they are more usually preceded by a gradual deterioration in control, which may not be noticed until it is quite advanced. A few patients, probably around 15-20%, will be unaware of moderate changes in their airflow obstruction even when these occur acutely; these patients are at particular risk of an acute exacerbation without warning. They should be encouraged to take regular peak flow recordings and enter them on a diary card to permit them to see trends in peak flow measurements and react to exacerbations at an early stage before there is any change in their symptoms.

Written asthma action plans

Mini peak flow meters are inexpensive and have an important role in educating patients about their asthma. Simply giving out a peak flow meter, however, has little benefit. Using home recordings, the doctor or nurse and patient can work together to develop plans with criteria that indicate the need for a change in treatment, a visit to the doctor, or emergency admission to hospital. This management plan should be written down for the patient and should be reviewed periodically. The peak flow can help the patient to interpret the severity of symptoms and need for help. It should be based on the patient's best known peak flow value.

It has not been possible to show an effect on the control of asthma or hospital admission from the use of a peak flow meter alone, but a written personal asthma action plan supported by regular follow-up does improve control. These have been shown to reduce emergency attendances and hospital admissions and improve lung function. They should show the

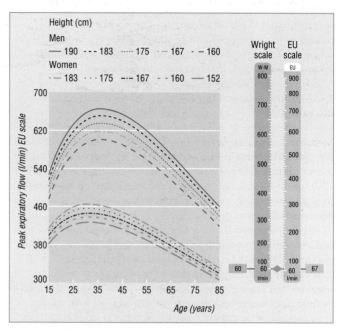

Earlier mini-Wright and Wright peak flow meters over-read at lower flow rates and are non-linear. Peak flow meters meeting the new European Union standard EN 13826 with an accurate peak flow measurement are available. Normal values for peak flow are shown on the left and the previous linear scale and compared with the accurate new scale for the mini-Wright peak shown on the right. Normal values are shown on the left, the range is such that readings up to 100 l/min lower than predicted are within normal limits for men. The equivalent figure is 85 l/min for women (values derived from Caucasian populations). Adapted from Nunn AJ, Gregg I. *BMJ* 1989;298:1068-70

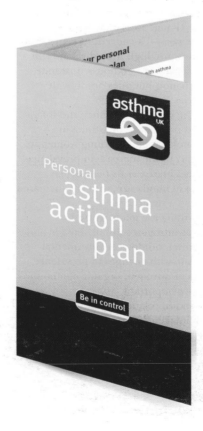

Asthma UK produces a self a management card which can be completed for each patient (Asthma UK) (see Appendix on p.63)

patient what to do, when to do it, for how long, and when further medical advice is needed.

Responsiveness to bronchodilators

Responses to bronchodilators are easy to measure in the clinic or surgery. Reversibility is often used to establish the diagnosis of asthma or to find out which is the most effective bronchodilator. Because of the variability in asthma, airflow obstruction may not be present at the time of testing. Reversibility is relatively specific but not very sensitive as a diagnostic test in patients with mild asthma.

Measuring reversibility

Reversibility is usually assessed by recording the best of three peak flow measurements and repeating the measurements 15-30 minutes after the patient has inhaled two or more doses of a β agonist—salbutamol or terbutaline—from a metered dose inhaler or dry powder system. The method of inhalation should be supervised and the opportunity taken to correct the technique or change to a different inhalation device if necessary. The 95% confidence intervals for a change in peak flow rate on such repetitions are around 60 l/min, and it is usual to look for a change in peak flow of 20% and 60 l/min. Reversibility can also be assessed in response to nebulised bronchodilator or a course of oral or inhaled steroid.

When forced expiratory volume in one second (FEV_1) is the measurement used, a change of 200 ml is outside the variability of the test. Such changes suggest asthma rather than COPD. A standard dose of a β agonist can be combined with an anticholinergic agent—ipratropium bromide. These agents are slower to act than β agonists, and their effect should be assessed 40-60 minutes after inhalation.

When there is severe obstruction and reversibility is limited, application of strict reversibility criteria may be correct for diagnosis but inappropriate for the purpose of determining treatments. Any response may be worth while so attention should be paid to subjective responses and improvement of exercise tolerance together with results of other tests of respiratory function. Reversibility shown by other tests, such as those of lung volumes or trapped gas volumes, without changes in peak flow or FEV_1 are more likely to occur in patients with COPD than in those with asthma.

Peak flow variation

Characteristic of asthma is a cyclical variation in the degree of airflow obstruction throughout the day. The lowest peak flow values occur in the early hours of the morning and the highest occur in the afternoon. To see the pattern a peak flow meter should be used at least twice and up to four times a day. Possible reasons for this variation include diurnal variation in adrenaline, vagal activity, cortisol, airway inflammation, and changes in β_2 receptor function.

Diurnal variation

Documentation of diurnal variation by recording measurements from a peak flow meter shows typical diagnostic patterns in many patients. The timing of the measurements should be recorded, otherwise typical variations can be obscured by later readings at the weekend or on days away from work or school. Variation has been calculated in several different ways. Amplitude % best is calculated as (highest−lowest)/highest × 100. Amplitude % best of 20% on three days of two consecutive weeks is likely to mean that asthma is present, but changes smaller than this do not exclude asthma.

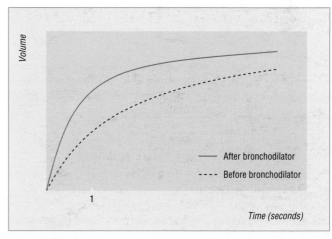

Reversibility in asthma is shown by change in FEV_1 on spirometry

Further review—Decisions about treatment from single dose studies should be backed up by further objective and subjective measurements during long term treatment. Responses to bronchodilators are not necessarily consistent, and, in some patients, changes after single doses in the laboratory may not predict the responses to the same drug over more prolonged periods

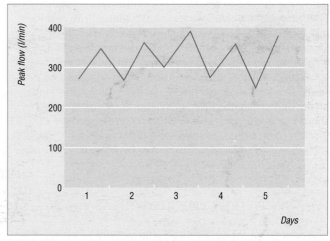

Diurnal percentage variation in peak flow readings. Amplitude percentage best is >20% each day ((highest−lowest)/highest × 100)

In people without asthma there is a small degree of diurnal variation with the same timing.

Nocturnal attacks

People with asthma commonly complain of waking at night. Large studies in the UK suggest that more than half of those with asthma have their sleep disturbed by an attack more than once a week. Questions about sleep disturbance by breathlessness and cough should be asked routinely in consultations with patients. Deaths from asthma are also more likely to occur in the early hours of the morning.

Exercise testing

The provocation test most often used in the United Kingdom is a simple exercise test. Exercise testing is a safe, simple procedure and may be useful when the diagnosis of asthma is in doubt. Patients without asthma do not develop bronchoconstriction on exercise; indeed they usually show a small degree of bronchodilation during the exercise itself. When baseline lung function is low, provocation testing is unnecessary for diagnosis as reversibility can be shown by bronchodilatation.

Exercise testing and the recording of diurnal variations are used when the history suggests asthma but lung function is normal when the patient is seen.

Testing outdoors

The exercise is best done outside because breathing cold dry air intensifies the response. The characteristic asthmatic response is a fall in peak flow of more than 15% several minutes after the end of exercise. About 90% of asthmatic children will show a drop in peak flow in response to exercise. Once the peak flow rate has fallen by 15% the bronchoconstriction should be reversed by inhalation of a bronchodilator. Late reactions about six hours after challenge are unusual, so, unlike challenge with an allergen, patients do not need to be kept under observation for late responses after the initial response has been reversed. Such tests are best avoided if the patient has ischaemic heart disease, but there is no reason why peak flow measurements should not be included during supervised exercise testing for coronary artery disease when this is appropriate.

Other types of challenge

The exercise test relies on changes in temperature and in the osmolality of the airway mucosa. Other challenge tests that rely on similar mechanisms include isocapnic hyperventilation; breathing cold, dry air; and osmotic challenge with nebulised distilled water or hypertonic saline. These are, however, laboratory based procedures whereas the simple exercise test for asthma can be done at any clinic or surgery.

Bronchodilators and sodium cromoglicate should be stopped at least six hours before the exercise test and long acting oral or inhaled bronchodilators and β antagonists should be stopped for at least 24 hours. Prolonged use of inhaled corticosteroids reduces responses to exercise, but these are not usually stopped before testing because the effect takes days or weeks to wear off.

Airway hyperresponsiveness

Other common forms of non-specific challenge to the airways are the inhalation of methacholine and histamine. These tests produce a range of responses, usually defined as the dose of the challenging agent necessary to produce a drop in the FEV of 20%. This is calculated by giving increasing doses until the FEV

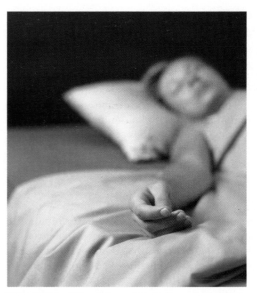

The lowest peak flow values occur in the early hours of the morning. With permission of Cristina Pedrazzini/Science Photo Library

An exercise test may consist of baseline peak flow measurements, then six minutes of vigorous supervised exercise such as running, followed by peak flow measurements for 30 minutes afterwards

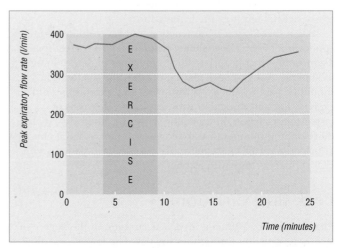

Decrease in peak expiratory flow rate in response to exercise

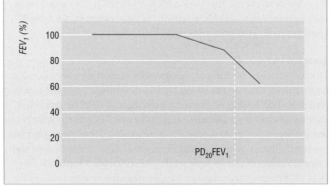

Low dose of histamine or methacholine

drops below 80% of the baseline measurement, then drawing a line to connect the last two points above and below a 20% drop and taking the dose at the point on this line equivalent to a 20% drop in FEV_1. Nearly all patients with asthma show increased responsiveness, whereas patients with hay fever and not asthma form an intermediate group.

This responsiveness of patients with asthma has been associated with the underlying inflammation in the airway wall. Such non-specific bronchial challenge is performed as an outpatient procedure in hospital respiratory function units. It is a safe procedure, providing it is monitored carefully and not used in the presence of moderately severe airflow obstruction.

Airway muscle is increased in asthma. There are smooth muscle growth factors in asthmatic airways and the smooth muscle cells themselves seem to respond differently.

Hyper-responsiveness may occur in people without asthma and in those with COPD. It would be unusual, however, to sustain the diagnosis of asthma in a patient with normal airway responsiveness on no treatment.

Degree of responsiveness

The degree of responsiveness is associated with the severity of the airways disease. It can be reduced by strict avoidance of known allergens. Drugs such as corticosteroids reduce responsiveness through their effect on inflammation in the wall of the airway, but they do not usually return reactivity to the normal range. Use of a bronchodilator is followed by a temporary reduction while the mechanisms of smooth muscle contraction are blocked.

Specific airway challenge

Challenge with specific agents to which a patient is thought to be sensitive must be done with caution. The initial dose should be low, and, even so, reactions may be unpredictable. Early narrowing of the airway by contraction of smooth muscle occurs within the first 30 minutes, and there is often a "late response" after four to eight hours.

The late response may be followed by poorer control of the asthma and greater diurnal variation for days or weeks afterwards. The late response is thought to be associated with release of mediators and attraction of inflammatory cells to the airways. It has been used in drug development as a more suitable model for clinical asthma than the brief early response.

Challenges with specific allergens are used mostly for the investigation of occupational asthma, but they should be restricted to experienced laboratories. Patients should be supervised for at least eight hours after challenge.

Skin tests

In skin prick tests a small amount of the test substance is introduced into the superficial layers of the epidermis on the tip of a small needle. The tests are painless, just causing temporary local itching. More general reactions are theoretically possible but extremely rare. Most young people with asthma show a range of positive responses to common environmental allergens such as house dust mite, pollens, and animal dander. A weal 3 mm larger than the negative control that develops 15 minutes after a skin prick test suggests the presence of specific IgE antibody; the results correlate well with those of in vitro tests for IgE such as the radioallergosorbent test (RAST), which is more expensive but may be helpful in difficult cases in the presence of widespread asthma.

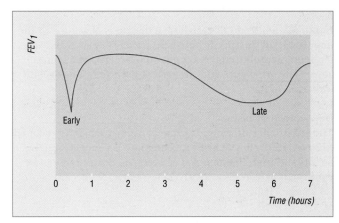

Drop in FEV_1 in a bronchial reactivity test

Bronchial reactivity is an important epidemiological and research tool. In clinical practice its use varies widely between countries. It is most useful where there are difficult diagnostic problems such as persistent cough

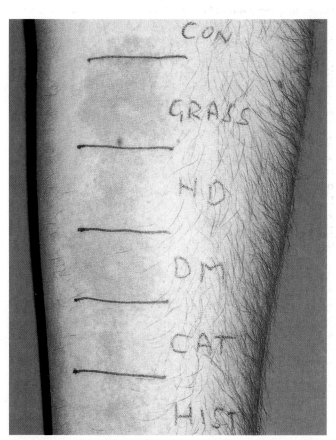

Skin prick tests. This patient is being exposed to a range of common allergens

Atopy

Positive skin tests do not establish a diagnosis of asthma or the importance of the specific allergens used. They show only the tendency to produce IgE to common allergens confirming atopy. The prevalence and strength of positive results decline with age.

Importance of history

The importance of allergic factors in asthma is best ascertained from a careful clinical history, taking into account seasonal factors and trials of avoidance of allergens. Suspicions can be confirmed by skin tests, RAST, or, less often, by specific inhalation challenge.

Conclusions

Although positive results to skin tests do not incriminate the allergen as a cause of the patient's asthma, it would be rare for an inhalant to be important in asthma with a negative result. The results do, however, rely on the quality of the agents used in testing and will be negative if antihistamines or leukotriene receptor antagonists are being taken. Bronchodilators and corticosteroids have no appreciable effect on immediate skin prick test results.

Differential diagnosis

The difficulty in breathing that is characteristic of asthma may be described as a constriction in the chest that suggests ischaemic cardiac pain. Nocturnal asthma that causes the patient to be woken from sleep by breathlessness may be confused with the paroxysmal nocturnal dyspnoea of heart failure.

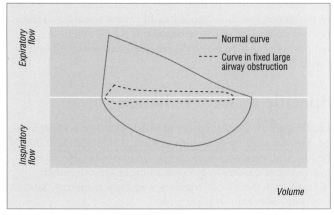

Flow volume curve

Asthma and COPD

After some years, particularly when it is severe, asthma may lose some or all of its reversibility. COPD, usually caused by cigarette smoking, may show appreciable reversibility, which can make it quite difficult to be sure of the correct diagnosis in older patients with partially reversible obstruction. The pathological changes in the airway are different in asthma and COPD.

In practice, however, bronchodilators are given and corticosteroids often used to establish the best airway function that can be achieved. Inhaled corticosteroids are much more important in asthma treatment than in COPD. When there is reversibility to bronchodilators and any doubt whether the diagnosis might be asthma, inhaled corticosteroids should be part of the treatment.

Non-asthmatic wheezing

Other causes of wheezing, such as obstruction of the large airways, occasionally produce problems in diagnosis. This may be the case with foreign bodies, particularly in children, or with tumours that gradually obstruct the trachea or main airways in adults. The noise produced is often a single pitched wheeze on inspiration and expiration rather than the multiple expiratory wheezes typical of widespread narrowing in asthma.

Appropriate x rays and flow volume loops can show the site of obstruction. On a flow volume curve a fixed low flow will be evident while on spirometry the volume time curve may be a straight line.

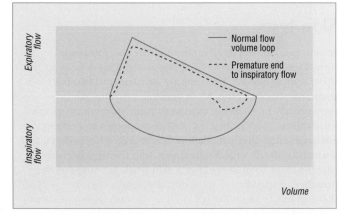

Vocal cord dysfunction: inspiratory flow stops prematurely because of glottic closure

Vocal cord dysfunction

Some patients have upper airway obstruction at the laryngeal level, produced apparently by dysfunction of the musculature of the vocal cords. The obstruction is most evident in inspiration and may show as premature termination of inspiration in the flow volume loop. The phenomenon seems to be more common in young women; it is often mistaken for, or coincident with, asthma and can be difficult to treat.

Further reading

- Gibson PG, Powell H. Written action plans for asthma: an evidence-based review of the key components. *Thorax* 2004;59:94-9.
- Share SA. Airway muscle in asthma is not just more of the same. *N Engl J Med* 2004;351:531-2.

4 Clinical course

Growing out of asthma

Parents of asthmatic children are usually concerned about whether their child will "grow out" of asthma. Most wheezy children improve during their teens, but the outlook depends to some extent on the severity of their early disease.

Over half the children whose wheezing is infrequent will be free of symptoms by the time they are 21, but of those with frequent troublesome wheezing, only 20% will be symptom-free at 21, although 20% will be substantially better. In 15% of patients, asthma becomes more troublesome in early adult years than it was in childhood. Even if there is prolonged remission lasting several years, symptoms may return later. In a New Zealand study wheezing was persistent in 14.5% of children up to the age of 26, while 12.4% wheezed in childhood, remitted, and then relapsed by 26. After months free from symptoms, biopsy studies show that the airway epithelium may still be inflamed and airway responsiveness to methacholine and histamine may remain abnormally high. This suggests that the underlying tendency to be asthmatic remains.

Likelihood of remission

Asthma is less likely to go into remission in patients with a strong family history of atopy or a personal history of other atopic conditions, low respiratory function, onset after the age of 29, and frequent attacks. More boys than girls are affected by asthma but the girls do less well during adolescence and by adulthood the sex ratio is equal. Most of those who do grow out of asthma are left with no residual effects other than the risk of recrudescence. Smoking increases the likelihood of persistence, while an early onset is predictive of relapse. In those with persistent asthma through childhood, results of respiratory function tests are significantly poorer. Chest deformities are uncommon and occur only when there is severe intractable disease.

Adult height

Although puberty may be delayed, the final adult height of children with asthma is usually normal unless they have received long term treatment with systemic or high dose inhaled corticosteroids.

Prognosis in adults

Asthma in adults often shows less spontaneous variation than it does in children. Wheezing is more persistent, and there is less association with obvious precipitating factors other than infections. The chances of a sustained remission are also lower than in children. Smokers with increased bronchial reactivity are particularly at risk of developing chronic airflow obstruction, and it is vital that people with asthma do not smoke. When there are known precipitating agents that can be avoided—such as animals or occupational factors—then sustained removal of these can reduce bronchial reactivity. The avoidance of contact with known allergens can decrease the inflammation in the airway wall and thus reduce responses to non-specific agents, including cigarette smoke, cold air, and dust. It can lead to an improvement in the control and the progress of the asthma.

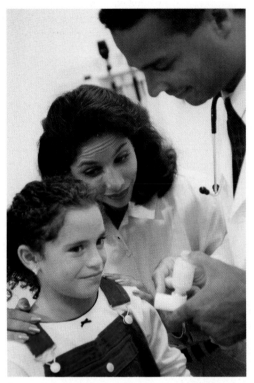

Parents hope that their children's asthma will improve as they get older

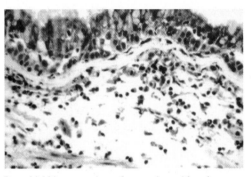

Bronchial biopsy specimen from patient with asthma showing eosinophilia and increased basement membrane (courtesy of Chris Corrigan)

Asthma: things to avoid

- Known allergens
- Active and passive cigarette smoking
- Areas of high pollution (particularly avoid exercising at times of high air pollution)
- β blockers
- Aspirin and non-steroidal anti-inflammatory drugs
- Obesity

The reversibility of airway obstruction in asthma is not always maintained throughout life. Those with more severe asthma are most likely to go on to develop irreversible airflow obstruction. It is likely that this progression to irreversibility is related to persistent inflammation of the wall of the airway, which leads to permanent damage through remodelling of the airway wall. Suitable prolonged prophylaxis reduces the inflammation, and most chest physicians act on the belief that this will reduce the likelihood of long term damage and eventual irreversibility. There are few prolonged studies to prove or disprove this contention, but the benefits of anti-inflammatory prophylaxis are well established in the short term, and it seems prudent to follow this practice.

A few studies on the introduction of inhaled corticosteroids give some hope that treatment can affect the clinical course. The degree of impairment in lung function when patient started inhaled steroids was greatest in those with the longest history of symptoms, suggesting that more prolonged untreated disease may lead to irreversible change. Delayed onset of inhaled steroids in one study comparing β agonists and steroids seemed to reduce the potential benefit of the steroids. Set against these studies are the changes seen at the end of trials of inhaled steroids. Bronchial responsiveness and lung function seem to return to baseline rapidly when treatment was stopped.

This is an important topic for further study, with implications for when to start inhaled steroids; the relative position in treatment of bronchodilators, steroids, and other agents such as cromoglicate, theophylline, and leukotriene antagonists, the degree of control that is looked for, and the approach to treatment once control is achieved.

Deaths from asthma

Since the sharp temporary increase in mortality from asthma seen in some countries during the early 1960s there has been concern about the role of treatment in such deaths. The deaths in the 1960s have been attributed to cardiac stimulation caused by overuse of inhaled isoprenaline or to excessive reliance on its usual efficacy leading to delay in using appropriate alternative treatment when symptoms worsened. Isoprenaline as a bronchodilator has been superseded by safer β_2 stimulants.

After the peak in the 1960s, the number of deaths from asthma in the United Kingdom stabilised. In the late 1980s there was a suggestion of a gradual rise in mortality to about 2000 per year but statistics for the 1990s show a gradual decline. The figures are most reliable for the ages 5–34, and the most recent figures confirm a slight fall in mortality in the group. Confidential inquiries into deaths suggest that clinical management issues have reduced, whereas patients' factors such as compliance and psychosocial problems have become more important.

Need for rapid response

Investigation of the circumstances surrounding individual deaths generally finds evidence of undertreatment rather than excessive medication in such deaths. Doctors and patients underestimate the severity of attacks; the most important factor may be an apparent reluctance to take oral corticosteroids for severe episodes and to adjust treatment early during periods of deterioration. Nevertheless, about a quarter of deaths occur less than an hour after the start of an exacerbation. Patients who have such rapid deterioration are particularly vulnerable. If patients have deteriorated swiftly in the past they should have suitable treatment readily available, such as steroids and nebulised and injectable bronchodilators. Patients and their relatives must be confident in the use of their emergency

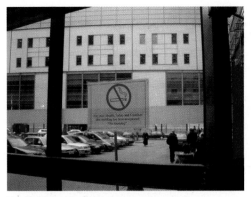

People with asthma must not smoke as they are at increased risk of developing chronic airflow obstruction. Smoking bans also help to improve and control the progress of asthma

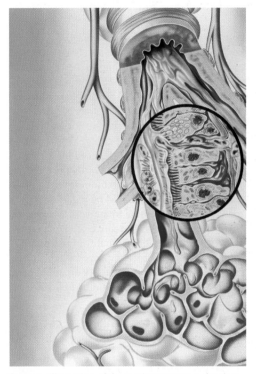

Cut away illustration of the respiratory system showing changes in severe asthma. A trigger such as an infection or allergen causes widespread narrowing of the airway through inflammation and bronchoconstriction. In addition, goblet cells produce excess sticky mucus, which can obstruct airways. Such mucus plugging is a prominent feature in fatal cases. With permission of John Bavosi/Science Photo Library

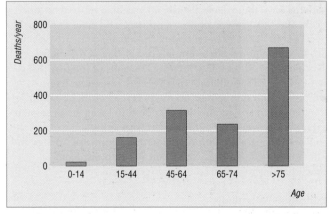

Overall numbers of deaths are greatest in the older age groups (Lung and Asthma Information Agency)

treatment and know how to obtain further help immediately.

Several centres have adopted the policy of maintaining a self admission service for selected patients. This avoids delay in admission to hospital and is a logical development of involving patients in the management of their own disease.

Diurnal variation

Some studies have shown that patients are particularly at risk after they have been discharged from intensive care or high dependency units to ordinary wards and after discharge from hospital. Problems often occur in the early hours of the morning at the nadir of the diurnal cycle. They may be related to premature tailing off of the initial intensive treatment because the measurements during the day have been satisfactory. Monitoring of peak flow will identify the instability of the asthma manifested by a large diurnal variability in peak flow. Adequate supervision and treatment must be maintained throughout these periods until control is restored.

British guideline on the management of asthma

Assessment and management in hospital have also been criticised. Asthma is a popular subject for audit according to the consensus guidelines of the British Thoracic Society (BTS) and the Scottish Intercollegiate Guidelines Network (SIGN). Studies have shown that initial assessment and treatment are satisfactory but that there are weaknesses in the exploration of reasons for an attack, establishment of adequate control before discharge, and arrangements for follow-up. Meeting the criteria of PEF >75% best or predicted, diurnal variability <25%, and establishment of a personalised management plan are the commonest problems in audits of asthma care. Every admission should be regarded as a failure of routine management. The usual treatment, compliance with therapy, and the existence and performance of management plans should be explored with the patient. Quality of treatment, readmission rates, and asthma control are improved when those with an interest in thoracic medicine supervise the inpatient care. Admission to hospital is an appropriate opportunity to involve a respiratory nurse specialist in the management.

Morbidity

Asthma causes considerable morbidity with persistent symptoms and loss of time from work and school. Repeated studies have shown that the aims of most guidelines are not met in a large proportion of patients. In milder disease (steps 1-3 of the BTS guidelines) the aim is control with no symptoms, no limitation of activity, and no adverse effects of treatment. This is achieved in less than half of patients, which suggests that the expectations of many doctors and patients are not high enough. Half of all patients have their sleep disturbed by asthma more than once a week, and this leads to poorer daytime performance. There has been a shift in the general approach to management, aiming to produce freedom from symptoms rather than a tolerable existence free of disabling attacks. The aims of the first three steps of the BTS guidelines involve virtual freedom from symptoms with minimal or no use of rescue bronchodilator. In children this would include freedom to take part in regular exercise. This requires a more aggressive approach early in the course of the disease with regular anti-inflammatory drugs and will, it is hoped, lead to a reduction in morbidity from exacerbations of asthma and long term damage.

Education of patients

Educating patients about their asthma and the use of treatment is an integral part of management. Internet sources from the

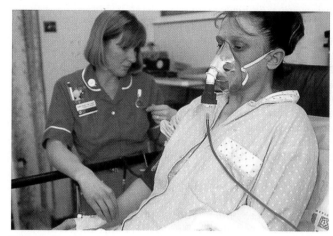

Woman with asthma in emergency department

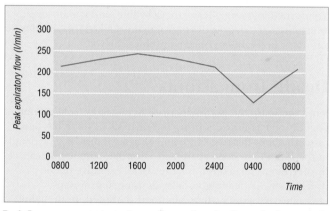

Peak flow measurements can be used to confirm the diagnosis of nocturnal asthma. Decreases in the early hours are associated with disturbed sleep and daytime tiredness

Categories of drug used in asthma	
Bronchodilators	**Preventers**
• Inhaled β agonists	• Inhaled corticosteroids
• Inhaled anticholinergics	• Sodium cromoglicate
• Theophyllines	• Nedocromil sodium
• Long acting β agonists	• Leukotriene receptor antagonists

lung and asthma information agency (www.laia.ac.uk) and Asthma UK (www.asthma.org.uk) provide useful reliable information. Patients forget much of what they are told in consultations and information should be backed up by written instructions. It is often helpful to produce these individually for each patient. Standard written information from asthma societies and other sources can be used as a backup, but a personal plan is preferable and can be produced from simple word processor templates. Patients are often confused about the differences between regular prophylaxis, such as inhaled corticosteroids or sodium cromoglicate, and the quickly effective inhaled bronchodilators used to treat acute attacks.

Regular use of a mini-peak flow meter allows the patient to participate more effectively in the understanding and treatment of the disease. Even with this information, though, many patients do not adhere to their prescribed regimen. Only half of all patients with asthma achieve 75% compliance with their prescribed treatment. This is true for all chronic conditions and shows the need for regular reinforcement (matching the information to the patients) and for further work in the area of education and compliance. Development of these management plans requires time, reinforcing and extending the information on repeat visits.

Asthma UK is a charity dedicated to improving the health and wellbeing of people in the UK whose lives are affected by asthma
Website: www.asthma.org.uk
Advice line: 08457 01 02 03
People can email an asthma nurse specialist at www.asthma.org.uk/adviceline

Further reading

- Bucknell CE, Slack R, Godley CC, Mackay TW, Wright SC. Scottish confidential inquiry in to asthma deaths (SCIAD) 1994-6. *Thorax* 2000;54:978-84.
- Campbell MJ, Cogman GR, Holgate ST, Johnston SL. Age specific trends in asthma mortality in England and Wales, 1983-95: results of an observational study. *BMJ* 1997;314:1439-41.
- Sears MR, Greene JM, Willan AR, Wiececk EM, Taylor DR, Flannery EM, et al. A longitudinal, population-based, cohort study of childhood asthma followed to adulthood. *N Engl J Med* 2003;349:14-22.

5 Precipitating factors

Bronchial hyperresponsiveness

The concept of increased reactivity of the airway to specific and non-specific stimuli is discussed in chapter 2. While inflammatory change in the airway wall is associated with increased reactivity, the underlying mechanisms of increased bronchial reactivity are uncertain. The sustained reactivity found in patients with asthma has been attributed to imbalance of autonomic control or other non-adrenergic, non-cholinergic plexuses, abnormal immunological and cellular responses, increased permeability of the epithelium, and intrinsic differences in the action of smooth muscle or its hypertrophy.

Non-specific stimuli

Airways in people with asthma are usually sensitive to non-specific stimuli such as dust and smoke. Laughing or coughing may provoke wheezing. Specific responses to agents such as pollen may lead to increased non-specific reactivity and symptoms of asthma for days or even weeks. Upper respiratory viral infections may lead to similar changes and may increase reactivity in people without asthma. In contrast, avoidance of exposure to known allergens may lead to improved control of asthma with reduced responses to other stimuli. Challenge to airways by specific allergens may induce late responses six to ten hours after exposure. Such late responses may mimic more closely the inflammatory changes caused by asthma that occur spontaneously. They lead to a subsequent rise in non-specific airway reactivity.

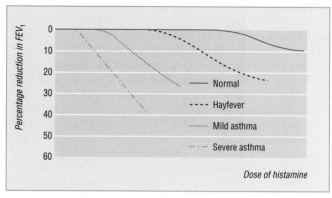

Bronchial reactivity is increased in people with asthma, particularly in those with severe disease

> The effect of exercise can be mimicked by breathing cold, dry air, whereas breathing warm, humid air—as in an indoor swimming pool—prevents the asthmatic response. In some patients, however, this picture is confused because they are sensitive to the chemical agents used in swimming pools

Exercise

Vigorous exercise produces narrowing of the airways in most people with asthma and, as described in chapter 2, can be used as a simple diagnostic test. Asthma during or after exercise is most likely to be a practical problem in children, in whom it may interfere with games at school. The type of exercise influences the response; most people find that swimming in warm indoor pools is the activity least likely to induce an attack. This observation has been explained by clinical studies showing the importance of cooling and drying of the airways during hyperventilation and exercise.

Drug prophylaxis

Many of the commonly used drugs protect against exercise induced asthma. Use of a short acting β agonist 15-30 minutes before exercise is usually effective and such treatments will normally allow a child to take part in games at school. Sodium cromoglicate and nedocromil sodium also block the response. Long acting β agonists and leukotriene receptor antagonists can prevent or minimise exercise induced asthma. It may be necessary to explain to teachers the use of the drugs and the objectives of the treatment.

Exercise itself is unlikely to have any major beneficial effect on asthma, but general fitness and weight control should be encouraged. A fit person can do a given task with less overall ventilation than an unfit one—hence the reduced likelihood of exercise-induced asthma. Asthma is quite compatible with a successful sporting career, as a number of athletes have testified, and the common inhaled asthma drugs, including inhaled

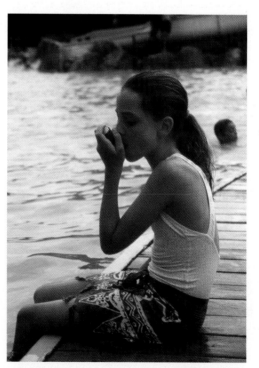

Premedication with a β stimulant or sodium cromoglicate usually allows children with asthma to participate in sports (Mark Clarke/Science Photo Library)

corticosteroids and long acting β agonists, are allowed in the regulations of most sporting bodies. The need for medication should be declared in advance. The number of athletes using medication for asthma has increased and the International Olympic Committee ask for medical confirmation and may require on site testing to show the need for medication. Various over the counter preparations for upper airway symptoms are not allowed.

Refractoriness

A second bout of exercise within an hour or so of the first is often less troublesome, a phenomenon known as refractoriness. The general benefits of warming up before exercise may therefore be greater for asthmatic athletes. Late asthmatic responses four to six hours after exposure to allergens are common, but they are rare and not troublesome after exercise.

Allergens in the home

Pets

The parents of children with asthma often worry about household pets. Cats cause the greatest problem, with allergens in saliva, urine, and dander, but most domestic animals can trigger asthma on occasions. Associated symptoms of conjunctivitis and rhinitis are common. People who have major problems with their asthma should be advised not to acquire any new pets.

When children are born into a family with a strong history of atopy, furry pets are best avoided. Pets already in residence should be kept out of bedrooms and off soft furnishings. If the animal seems to be a cause of serious symptoms, a trial separation should be organised. Animal allergens remain in the house long after the pet is removed so the pet should move out for a month or two; alternatively the patient could move out for a week or two. Unjustified removal of favourite pets without good reason may, however, provoke more serious problems from emotional upset.

The position is complicated by evidence that asthma is less common in children born to families with pets or domestic animals. This is connected with the maturation of the immune system from early exposure to allergens and infections.

Dust mites

The house dust mite, *Dermatophagoides pteronyssinus*, provides the material for the most common positive skin prick test in the UK. The main allergen is found in the mites' faecal pellets. The mites live off human skin scales and are widely distributed in bedding, furniture, carpets, and soft toys and thrive best in warm damp conditions. The expectation of a warm environment at home has increased the exposure of children to allergens and is likely to be an important element in the increased prevalence of asthma.

Change of environment

If patients move into environments that are completely free of house dust mites their symptoms improve. This can be achieved in the mountains of Switzerland or near to home, but less picturesque, in specially cleaned hospital wards without soft furnishings.

It is more difficult to reduce the numbers of mites sufficiently in the home. Regular cleaning of bedrooms and avoiding materials that are particularly likely to collect dust are sensible measures to keep down the antigenic load. Substantial reduction in mite antigen is possible by reducing the amount of soft furnishing and carpets, extensive cleaning, and the use of mattress covers made of materials such as

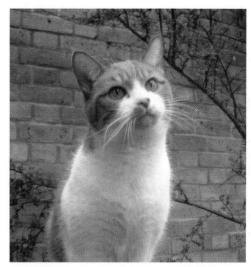

Cats are the most problematic domestic pet for people with asthma

---

Measures to control house dust mite

Though the effects are small, families who want to deal with house dust mites can try:
- Impervious covers on mattresses and soft furnishings
- Hard floors instead of carpets
- No soft toys in the bedroom
- Acaricides applied regularly to soft furnishings
- Washing bed clothes at high temperatures
- Damp dusting
- Dehumidification

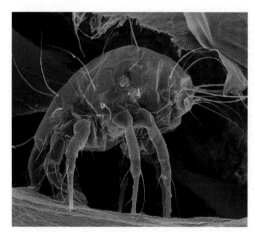

Light micrograph of dust mite (Steve Gshmeissner/Science Photo Library)

Cockroaches—recent studies have shown high levels of sensitivity to cockroach allergen in some areas. These levels are around 50% in institutions and lower socioeconomic groups

Gortex, which are impermeable to mites. Acaricides, or even applications of liquid nitrogen to mattresses, can produce a temporary reduction. Vacuum cleaners fitted with fine filters may help, in combination with measures that deal with reservoirs of antigen in sites such as mattresses. Although these measures reduce mite numbers they have little effect on control of asthma, probably because they do not produce enough of a sustained reduction in house dust mite antigen. Desensitisation to house dust mites may be of some use in children.

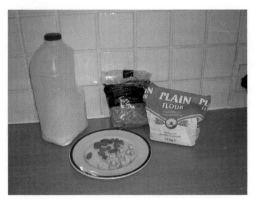

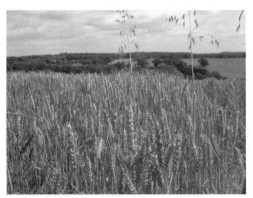

Food allergy is sometimes a factor in asthma

Food allergy

Food allergy causes eczema and gastrointestinal symptoms more often than asthma, but some striking cases do occur. Exclusion diets have generally given disappointing results in asthma; immediate skin prick tests and radioallergosorbent tests are less useful than for inhaled allergens. Most serious cases of asthma induced by food intolerance are evident from a carefully taken history, so elaborate diets are not warranted. When there is doubt, suspicions can be confirmed by excluding the agent from the diet or by controlled exposure.

Intolerance to food does not always indicate an allergic mechanism. Reactions may be related to pharmacological mediators such as histamine or tyramine in the food. They may be produced by food additives such as the yellow dye tartrazine, which is added to a wide range of foods and medications. When there is a specific allergy to foodstuffs, the most likely to be implicated are milk, eggs, nuts, and wheat. Management can be difficult because of the use of nuts in a wide range or products.

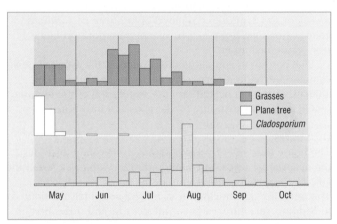

Exposure to specific pollens and spores can be seasonal

Pollens and spores

Seasonal asthma, often together with rhinitis and conjunctivitis, is usually associated with grass pollens, which are most common during June and July. Less common in the UK is precipitation of asthma by tree pollens, much of which is produced between February and May, and mould spores from *Cladosporium* and *Alternaria*, which abound in July and August. Complete avoidance of such widespread pollens is impractical.

Hyposensitisation
The effectiveness of hyposensitisation is debatable. It is generally unnecessary because inhaled drugs usually produce adequate control and are simple to use. The strong placebo effect, allergic reactions to hyposensitisation, and the occasional death must also be taken into account in assessing its value. Some studies show some benefits and advances in allergen production and manipulation may lead to greater future use.

Seasonal variations in allergens

Legend: ■ Grasses □ Plane tree □ *Cladosporium*

May — Jun — Jul — Aug — Sep — Oct

Allergic bronchopulmonary aspergillosis

Some people with asthma develop sensitivity to the spores of *Aspergillus fumigatus*, which is a common fungus particularly partial to rotting vegetation. Allergic bronchopulmonary aspergillosis is associated with eosinophilia in blood and sputum, rubbery brownish plugs of mucus containing fungal hyphae, and proximal bronchiectasis. Areas of consolidation and collapse may be visible in the chest x ray film, and each episode can lead to further bronchiectatic damage. The aspergillus skin test result will be positive and specific IgE will be found in the blood.

Individual episodes settle after treatment with corticosteroids, but if they are frequent and bronchiectasis is developing then long term oral corticosteroids may be

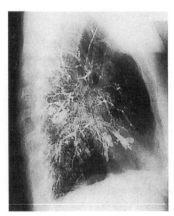

Bronchiectasis in a patient with allergic bronchopulmonary aspergillosis

appropriate. Antifungal imidazoles such as itraconazole may also reduce the frequency of attack.

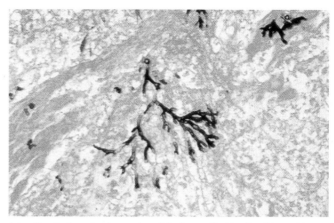

Aspergillus fumigatus hyphae and conidiophores (fruiting heads)

Features of allergic bronchopulmonary aspergillosis

- Difficult asthma
- Chest x ray changes, consolidation, or collapse
- Brownish rubbery sputum plugs
- Eosinophilia
- Specific IgE against aspergillus
- Positive result on aspergillus skin test
- Proximal bronchiectasis

Occupational asthma

The importance of occupational asthma is increasingly being recognised. Some estimates suggest that up to 10% of cases of adult asthma have an occupational origin and over 200 precipitating agents have been reported. People with asthma should avoid occupations where they are likely to be exposed to large quantities of non-specific stimuli such as dust and cold air. An occupational element should always be considered, particularly with adult onset asthma

Definition

Occupational asthma is officially recognised as an industrial disease and is subject to compensation. It is defined as asthma that "develops after a variable period of symptomless exposure to a sensitising agent at work" (www.occupationalasthma.com/). Fourteen agents are currently recognised for compensation, and this list is kept under regular review. Agents such as proteolytic enzymes and laboratory animals are particularly likely to produce problems in atopic people, whereas isocyanate asthma is not related to atopic status. In some studies potent agents such as platinum salts have produced asthma in up to half of those who are exposed to them.

Diagnosis

Increased bronchial reactivity provoked by occupational agents may persist long after the person is no longer exposed. Regular peak flow recordings are once again an important diagnostic tool and usually show a distinct relation to time at work, but the association may not be obvious because the timing of the responses is variable. Reactions may occur soon after arrival at work, be delayed until later in the day, or come on slowly over several days. In some cases a weekend away from work may not be long enough for lung function to return to normal and absence for a week or two may be necessary. Initial investigations include exploration of potential agents at work and recording peak flow patterns every two or four hours at and away from work. Further investigation may require specific challenge testing in an experienced laboratory.

Management

Awareness and early detection are important as occupational asthma is the one area where appropriate management can affect the natural course of the disease. The first approach to management should be to try to adjust the conditions at work that produced the sensitisation. If this is not possible the patient may be able to continue working with a mask to provide filtered air. If these measures fail and simple inhaled treatment is inadequate then a change of job will be necessary. It is advisable to try to obtain, with the patient's consent, the cooperation of any occupational health staff in the workplace at an early stage. Employers are requested to report cases under the Reporting of Injuries, Diseases and Dangerous Occurrences Regulations (RIDDOR).

Some causes of occupational asthma

Chemicals
- Isocyanates
- Platinum salts
- Epoxy resins
- Aluminium
- Hair sprays
- Azodicarbonamide (plastic blowing)

Vegetable sources
- Wood dusts
- Dust meal such as flour from grains
- Coffee beans
- Colophony (solders)
- Cotton, flax, hemp dust
- Castor bean dust
- Latex

Enzymes
- Trypsin
- *Bacillus subtilis*

Animals
- Laboratory rodents
- Shellfish
- Larger mammals
- Locusts
- Grain weevil, mites

Drug manufacture
- Penicillins
- Piperazine
- Salbutamol
- Cimetidine
- Isphaghula
- Ipecacuanha

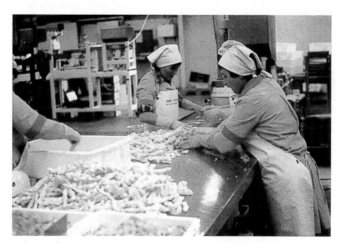

A cluster of wheezing and rhinitis occurred on this prawn processing line. High pressure hoses (used to free prawns from the shells) had created aerosols containing crustacean protein. From Snashall D, Patel D (eds) *ABC of Occupational and Environmental Medicine*, 2nd ed, Blackwell Publishing, 2003

Within industry, problems arise most often from exposure to glutaraldehyde used in disinfection procedures, latex from gloves and proteins in the urine of small animals in laboratory technicians and researchers.

Drug induced asthma

Two main groups of drugs are responsible for most cases of drug-induced asthma: β blocking agents and prostaglandin synthetase inhibitors such as aspirin.

β blockers

β blocking agents usually induce bronchoconstriction when they are given to patients with asthma, and this may happen even when they are given in eye drops. Relatively selective β blockers, such as atenolol and metoprolol, are less likely to cause severe irreversible asthma, but the whole group of β blocking drugs should be avoided in patients who already have asthma. For patients with hypertension, diuretics, angiotensin converting enzyme inhibitors, or calcium antagonists are suitable alternatives. When asthma is produced by β blockade, large doses of β stimulants are necessary to reverse it, particularly with less selective β blockers. Fortunately, cardiac side effects of treatment with β stimulants are not a problem because they are also inhibited by the β blockade.

Prostaglandin synthetase inhibitors

Salicylates provoke severe narrowing of the airways in a small group of adults with asthma. About 2-3% of people with asthma have a history of sensitivity to aspirin, but around 20% have some sensitivity on provocation testing. Once such a reaction has been noted these patients should avoid contact with aspirin or non-steroidal anti-inflammatory agents, which usually produce the same effects. The mechanism is probably related to changes in arachidonic acid metabolism with increased production of leukotrienes. Milder salicylate sensitivity can be shown more often on routine testing, particularly in adults with asthma and nasal polyps.

Ibuprofen is available without prescription and has the same effects. Patients are often unaware of the presence of salicylate in common compound preparations and cold cures. When salicylate sensitivity is suspected the patient should be asked to check carefully the contents of any such medication they take. When salicylate reactions occur it may be possible to induce tolerance by carefully building up from small oral doses. This should be done only in experienced units.

Iatrogenic effects

Occasionally, drugs used to treat asthma can themselves be responsible for provoking bronchoconstriction. Such paradoxical effects have been described with aminophylline, ipratropium bromide, sodium cromoglicate, β agonists in infants, and propellants or contaminants from the valve apparatus in metered dose inhalers.

Hypotonic solutions can cause bronchoconstriction in people with asthma, and nebuliser solutions should be made up with normal saline rather than water. Preservatives in some nebuliser solutions have also produced narrowing of the airways.

Emotional factors

Psychological factors can play an important part in asthma. On their own they do not produce asthma in people without an underlying susceptibility, but in the laboratory emotional factors and expectation influence the bronchoconstrictor responses to

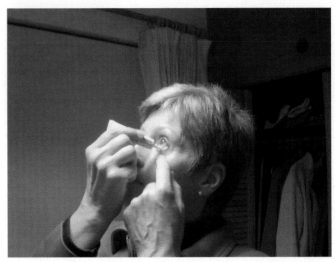

Absorption of β blockers through the conjunctive can precipitate asthma

---

Drugs that can induce asthma

- β blockers (including eye drops)
- Aspirin and non-steroidal anti-inflammatory drugs
- Inhaled asthma drugs
- Nebuliser solutions, hypotonic or with preservatives
- Angiotensin converting enzyme inhibitors

In epidemiological studies both aspirin and paracetamol have been associated with increased mortality from asthma. Cox 2 inhibitors seem to be safe in those who are sensitive to aspirin

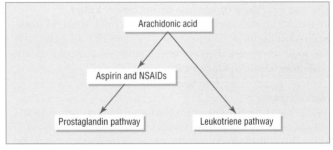

Aspirin blocks prostaglandin synthetase activity and sends arachidonic acid metabolism down the leukotriene pathway. This is likely to be the basis of aspirin induced asthma

various specific and non-specific stimuli and the bronchodilator responses to treatment. Stress and emotional disturbance are factors that must be taken into account in the overall management of patients with asthma. In children the position is complicated by the emotional responses of their parents.

Confidence and relaxation

Emotional problems are more likely to occur when control of asthma is poor, and these problems are best managed by increasing the confidence of patients and relatives with adequate explanation and control of the asthma. It is particularly important that patients know exactly what to do during an acute exacerbation. More specific measures such as relaxation, yoga, hypnotherapy, and acupuncture have been investigated. Some trials have shown beneficial effects, and some patients obtain considerable help from relaxation treatment. It can be dangerous, however, if conventional medicines are neglected when alternative approaches are adopted.

Asthma associated with emotional outbursts such as laughing and crying may be related to the response of hyper-reactive airways to deep inspirations or to inhalation of cold, dry air rather than to the emotion itself. People with a tendency to be manipulative may, of course, use a condition such as asthma for their own purposes just as they might use any other chronic disease.

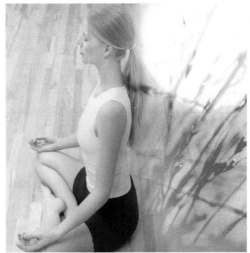

Relaxation can be of help, but it is not a substitute for drug therapy (photos.com)

Pollution

Personal air pollution with cigarette smoke worsens asthma; active and passive smoking provoke narrowing of the airways.

Air quality

There has been increased interest in environmental pollution in recent years. Though the inner city smogs disappeared after the introduction of the Clean Air Act 1956, high levels of ozone, sulphur dioxide, oxides of nitrogen, and particulate matter develop in certain areas and in particular climatic conditions. Combinations of high temperature, humidity, and heavy traffic can cause levels of these pollutants above those in the guidelines of the World Health Organization. Increased symptoms and admissions have been linked to levels of nitrogen dioxide and sulphur dioxide and, in some studies, ozone. High levels of small particulate matter are associated with increased mortality from cardiorespiratory diseases. People with asthma should be aware of measures of air quality.

Weather

Climatic conditions such as the pressure and humidity associated with thunderstorms can provoke asthma. The conditions may increase the concentrations of fungal and pollen spores at ground level as they are brought down from higher levels of the atmosphere. The spores rupture to produce particles of respirable size.

Indoor environment

Indoor pollution can also cause problems. Oxides of nitrogen are produced from heating and cooking. Formaldehyde and moulds and other biological compounds may occur in dwellings. Concentrations of nitrogen dioxide found in the home may increase airway responses to common allergens such as house dust mite, and the average UK citizen spends 85-90% of their time indoors.

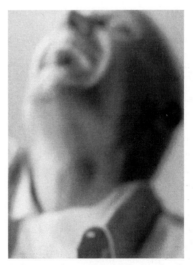

Asthma can be associated with emotional outbursts such as laughing

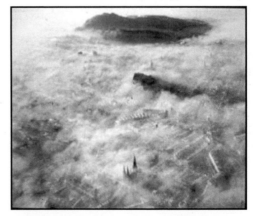

Air quality can be poor, especially in large cities. From Florida-James G, Donaldson K, Stone V. Sports performance in a polluted evironment. In: Whyte GP, et al (eds) *ABC of Sports and Exercise Medicine*, 3rd ed. Blackwell Publishing, 2005

Asthma and pregnancy

The control of asthma during pregnancy can change, but the effect is variable. About a third of patients improve, a third worsen, and a third continue unchanged. The effect may vary in different pregnancies in the same woman. Breathlessness may be more pronounced in late pregnancy as the diaphragmatic movement is limited even without any change in airflow obstruction.

Drug treatment during pregnancy

There is a natural anxiety about the use of drugs during pregnancy. Fortunately the usual asthma treatments of inhaled β agonists, and inhaled and oral corticosteroids have been shown to be safe. Leukotriene receptor antagonists are best avoided until more safety information is available. Control and supervision of asthma should be improved during pregnancy to reduce the likelihood of an acute exacerbation. Acute attacks should be treated vigorously in the normal way. Severe asthma and hypoxia rather than treatments for asthma are the potential danger during pregnancy.

Further reading

- Gotzsche P, Johansen H, Schmidt L, Burr M. House dust mite control measures for asthma. *Cochrane Database Syst Rev* 2004;(4):CD001187.
- Wark P. Pathogenesis of allergic bronchopulmonary aspergillosis and an evidence based review of azoles in treatment. *Respir Med* 2004;98:915-23.

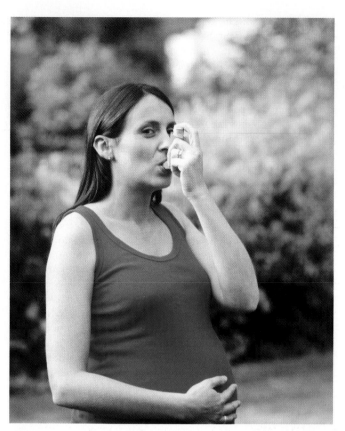

Women are naturally anxious about using drugs during pregnancy. With permission from Paul Whitehill/Science Photo Library

6 General management of acute asthma

Assessment of severity

The speed of onset of acute attacks of asthma varies. Some severe episodes come on over a period of minutes with no warning, although more often there is a background of deterioration over days or weeks. This period during which control of the asthma deteriorates tends to be longer in older patients. A good early guide to developing problems is the need to use bronchodilator inhalers more often than usual or finding that they are less effective.

Peak flow monitoring
Deterioration in control can also be detected by measurement of peak flow at home; a drop in the peak flow or an increase in the diurnal variation of peak flow provides evidence of instability. Detecting these changes allows a change of treatment while the decline is slow and before severe problems arise. Even if patients do not use their peak flow meter regularly it can be useful to confirm changes in symptoms.

Breathlessness
The most common symptom is breathlessness, and there is more likely to be a sensation of difficulty in inspiration than in expiration. Some patients have a poor appreciation of changes in the degree of their airflow obstruction and will complain of few symptoms until they have developed moderately severe asthma. They are more likely to develop severe asthma and are at particular risk during acute attacks. When such patients are identified they should be encouraged to use a peak flow meter regularly to provide objective evidence of their asthma control. For these patients regular monitoring of peak flow is particularly important. Some studies of patients who have had life threatening asthma show that patients with psychosocial problems, poor adherence to treatment, and high levels of denial are over-represented compared with those with good control.

As the severity of the asthma increases, breathlessness begins to interfere with simple functions. Exercise is limited and later, eating and drinking are difficult. In severe attacks it will be difficult for the patient to speak in full sentences without gasping for breath between words. Knowledge of the pattern of previous attacks is important as the progress is often broadly similar in subsequent episodes.

Patients must be taught to seek help early rather than late in an acute exacerbation; it is easier to step in and prevent deterioration into severe asthma than to treat a full blown attack. Patients and their families should all be confident about the management of exacerbations—not only regarding the immediate treatment but also about how and when to seek further help and hospital admission. These should all be discussed before the first acute attack of asthma.

Examination

Inability to speak will be obvious when the history is taken. Respiratory rate is a useful sign and should be counted accurately; a rate of ≥25 breaths per minute is a sign of severity Hypoxia severe enough to cause confusion occurs only in severe asthma and means that admission to hospital and

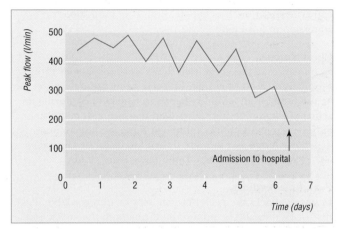

Gradual deterioration in peak flow in acute exacerbation

> All patients with asthma should be aware of what to do if they fail to get relief from their usual treatment. Patients and relatives should have a written action plan that should include trigger levels of peak flow as percentage of their best known or symptoms that require changes in treatment or consultation for further advice

---

Assessment of severity in asthma

Always err on the side of caution in assessment. In general, those with acute severe asthma or life threatening asthma should be referred to hospital. Other factors such as response to treatment, social circumstances, or other medical conditions may influence decisions about place of treatment. Outside hospital the following features can be used to assess severity:

Life threatening asthma (any one of):
- PEF <33% of best or predicted
- SaO_2 <92% as a feature of life threatening asthma
- Silent chest
- Cyanosis
- Feeble respiratory effort
- Bradycardia
- Dysrhythmia
- Hypotension
- Exhaustion
- Confusion
- Coma

Acute severe asthma
- PEF 33-50% of best or predicted
- Respiratory rate ≥25/min
- Heart rate ≥110/min
- Inability to talk in sentences without breaths

Moderate exacerbations
- PEF 50-75% of best or predicted
- No features of acute severe asthma

---

supplemental oxygen are needed urgently. The pulse rate is also a useful guide to severity: tachycardia >110 beats per minute is found in severe episodes, though this sign may be less reliable in elderly people, when pulse rates tend to remain low. In extremely severe attacks bradycardia may occur.

Pulsus paradoxus (a drop in systolic pressure of >10 mm Hg on inspiration) is a traditional measurement in acute asthma but is not useful in practice. Any evidence of circulatory embarrassment, such as hypotension, is an indication for admission to hospital.

Chest sounds

Examination of the chest itself shows a fast respiratory rate, overinflation, and wheezing. In severe acute asthma airflow may be too little for an audible wheeze, so a quiet chest during an acute attack is worrying rather than reassuring. It may also indicate a pneumothorax (although these are not common in acute asthma, and they are difficult to diagnose clinically; a chest x ray film must be taken if there is any doubt).

Peak flow readings

In severe attacks the peak flow rate may be unrecordable. Peak flow or FEV should be monitored throughout the attack and during recovery as they are reliable, simple guides to the effectiveness of treatment. Peak flow values are easier to interpret if the patient's usual or best readings are known.

Blood gases

An initial measurement of blood gases should be done in patients with asthma severe enough to warrant admission to hospital. Great care should be taken in obtaining arterial blood because some asthmatic patients who have had bad experiences of arterial puncture may delay attendance at hospital because of the memories of pain. In patients with mild attacks a pulse oximeter should be used in the accident and emergency department. If saturation is ≥93% while the patient is breathing air and he or she does not have signs of severe asthma, then blood gas measurement can be omitted. In more severe cases oxygen saturation by pulse oximeter can be used to assess progress after the first arterial gas measurement, provided the initial carbon dioxide tension was not raised and there is no sign of appreciable deterioration.

Hypoxia and hypercapnia

Some hypoxia is usual and responds to supplemental oxygen. An arterial oxygen tension of ≤8 kPa on air is a mark of severity. As long as the patient does not have COPD there is no need to limit the concentration of supplemental oxygen. The arterial carbon dioxide tension is usually low in acute asthma; occasionally it is high on admission, particularly in children, but quickly responds to treatment with a bronchodilator. Hypercapnia, however, is an alarming feature of acute asthma, and failure either to reduce carbon dioxide retention during the first hour or to prevent its development during treatment is an indication that mechanical ventilation must be considered. The final decision on this depends on the overall clinical state of the patient rather than on the blood gas measurement alone.

Where to treat acute asthma

An acute attack of asthma is frightening; transfer to hospital might exacerbate symptoms by producing anxiety, and reassurance that treatment is available to relieve the attack is an important part of the management. It is not possible to lay down strict criteria for admission to hospital. The features of severity discussed above should, however, be assessed.

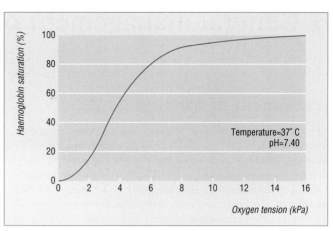

Normal oxyhaemoglobin dissociation curve. Saturation low enough to produce visible cyanosis is a sign of very severe asthma

In hospital blood gases provide extra information and PaO_2 <8 kPa or a normal $PaCO_2$ of 4.6-6.0 kPa (that is, not the low $PaCO_2$ expected in milder attacks) are also features of life threatening asthma

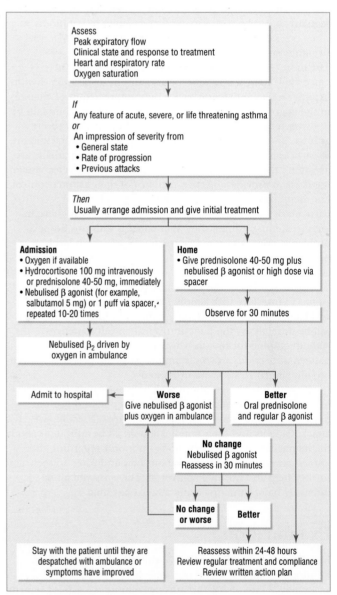

Treatment of acute severe asthma in general practice. Adapted from guidelines from the British Thoracic Society and Scottish Intercollegiate Guidelines Network

Most of the dangers of acute asthma come from a failure to appreciate the severity of an attack and the absence of suitable supervision and treatment to follow up the initial response.

Immediate improvement after the first nebuliser treatment may provide false reassurance, being followed quickly by the return of severe asthma, so continued observation is essential.

Initial treatment

It may be obvious on first seeing the patient that supplemental oxygen and hospital treatment are necessary. Treatment should be started while this is arranged. In less severe attacks initial treatment should be given and, if the response is inadequate, hospital admission should be arranged. If the initial response is adequate it may be possible to manage the patient at home if supervision is available. The primary treatment should then be followed up, usually by adequate bronchodilation and corticosteroids, and the response should be assessed by measurements of peak flow. The threshold for admission should be lowered if there has been a recent admission, previous severe attacks, poor patient perception of severity, or poor social support.

Dangers of undertreatment

Most deaths from asthma occur when the patient or doctor has failed to appreciate the severity of the attack. When there is any doubt it is safer to opt for vigorous treatment and admission to hospital. When treatment is given at home, the patient's condition must be assessed regularly and often until the exacerbation has settled. The reason for the acute exacerbation and the patient's response must always be reviewed.

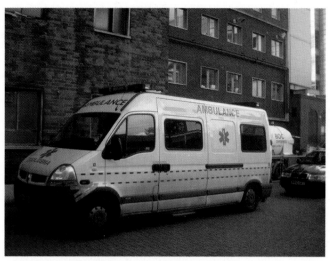

Appropriate treatment should be started before transfer to hospital, with nebulised bronchodilators and oxygen continued during transfer

British guideline on the management of asthma.
www.brit-thoracic.org.uk/docs/asthmafull.pdf

7 Treatment of acute asthma

The initial assessment of a patient with increased symptoms of asthma is very important. Most problems result from undertreatment and failure to appreciate severity. Monitor the peak flow rate and other signs before and after the first nebuliser treatment, and then as appropriate. In hospital, peak flow should be monitored at least four times a day for the duration of the stay. A flow chart for the management of asthma at home is shown in chapter 6 (p.26) and a flow chart for management in hospital is given on p.31. The various aspects of treatment are considered individually in this chapter.

β agonists

Adrenaline has been used in the treatment of asthma since just after the first world war. The specific short acting β_2 agonists such as salbutamol and terbutaline have replaced the earlier non-selective preparations for acute use. There are no great differences in practice between the commonly used agents. If long acting bronchodilators are used they can be continued during the attack.

Use and availability of nebulisers

In acute asthma, metered dose inhalers often lose their effectiveness. This is largely because of difficulties in the delivery of the drugs to the airways because of coordination problems and narrowing and occlusion of the airways.

An alternative method of giving them is necessary—usually by nebuliser or intravenously. A large volume spacer (for example, Nebuhaler or Volumatic) can be as effective as a nebuliser in most cases. Like the nebuliser it has the advantage of removing the need to coordinate inhaler actuation and breathing. There is little or no difference in the effectiveness of drugs that are nebulised or given intravenously in acute severe asthma, so nebulisation is generally preferable.

It is helpful for general practitioners to have nebulisers available for acute asthmatic attacks. In acute asthma, β_2 agonists are best given by nebulisers driven by oxygen as they may even worsen hypoxia slightly through an effect on the pulmonary vasculature. In general practice the use of oxygen as the driving gas is not usually practical. Domiciliary oxygen sets do not produce a flow rate adequate to drive most nebulisers, but, if available, they can be used with nasal cannulae during the nebulisation for a patient having an acute attack. Many ambulance staff are able to give nebulised drugs and oxygen during transfer to hospital.

In hospital, nebulisers used to treat asthmatic patients should be driven by oxygen unless the patient has COPD with carbon dioxide retention. The driving gas, flow rate, drug diluent, and volume of fill should be clearly written on the prescription chart. Dilutions should always be done with saline to avoid bronchoconstriction from nebulisation of hypotonic solutions. There is no real advantage of nebulisation with a machine capable of producing intermittent positive pressure.

For adults the initial dose should be 5 mg salbutamol or its equivalent. This should be halved if the patient has ischaemic heart disease. It is essential to continue the intensive treatment after the first response; many of the problems in acute asthma arise because of complacency after the initial response to the

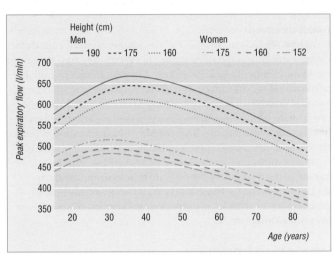

Predicted values for peak expiratory flow. Adapted from Nunn AJ, Gregg I. *BMJ* 1989; 298:1068-70

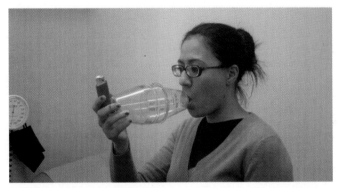

Attaching a spacer to a metered dose inhaler avoids the need for co-ordination between firing and inhalation

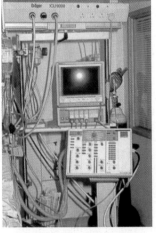

Acute attacks may require admission to an intensive care unit

first treatment. In severe attacks the nebulisation may need to be repeated every 15 to 30 minutes and can even be continuous.

Parenteral delivery

If nebulised drugs are not effective then parenteral treatment should be considered. A reasonable plan is to give a β_2 agonist the first time, combine with an anticholinergic drug for the second nebulisation, and move to intravenous bronchodilators if there is no improvement. If life threatening features such as a raised carbon dioxide tension, an arterial oxygen tension <8 kPa on oxygen, or a low pH are present, the intravenous agent should be used from the start.

The bronchodilator given parenterally in an acute attack can be a β_2 agonist or aminophylline. There is little to choose between them. If the patient has been taking theophylline and the blood concentration is not immediately available it is safer to use the β_2 agonist. Salbutamol or terbutaline can be given intravenously over 10 minutes or as an infusion, usually at 5-15 μg per minute. The adverse effects of tachycardia and tremor are much more common after intravenous injection than after nebulisation.

Anticholinergic agents

Ipratropium bromide is the only anticholinergic agent available in nebulised form in the UK. Nebulised ipratropium seems to be as effective as a nebulised β agonist in acute asthma. The dose of ipratropium is 500 μg, and there are no problems with increased viscosity of secretions or mucociliary clearance at such doses. Ipratropium starts working more slowly than salbutamol: the peak response may not occur for 30-60 minutes.

Adverse reactions such as paradoxical bronchoconstriction have been reported occasionally. These were related mainly to the osmolality of the solution or to the preservatives, and they have been corrected in the current preparations.

Although the combination of β stimulant and anticholinergic agents produces a greater effect than use of a single agent, the difference is small and β_2 agonists are sufficient for most patients. It is reasonable to start with a β_2 agonist alone and add ipratropium if the response to the first nebulisation is not considered adequate. If the initial assessment indicates that it is a very severe attack then the combination should be used from the start.

Methylxanthines

Aminophylline is an effective bronchodilator in acute asthma, but most studies have shown that it is no more effective than a β_2 agonist given by nebulisation or intravenously. There are more problems with its use than with nebulised drugs, and it should be reserved for patients with life threatening features or who have failed to respond to nebulised drugs. Toxic effects are common and can occur with drug concentrations in or just above the therapeutic range. Concentrations are difficult to predict from the dose given because of individual differences in metabolic rate and interactions with drugs such as nicotine, cimetidine, erythromycin, and ciprofloxacin.

The position is further complicated if patients are already taking oral theophyllines. The usual starting dose for intravenous aminophylline is 250 mg given over 20-30 minutes. If the patient has taken oral theophylline or aminophylline in the previous 24 hours and a blood concentration is not available then the initial dose should be omitted or halved. A continuous infusion is then given at a rate of 0.5 mg/kg/hour, though this dose should be reduce if the patient also has kidney or liver disease. If intravenous treatment is necessary for more

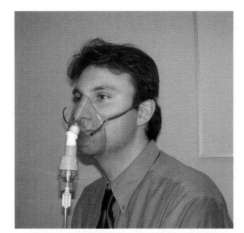

In acute asthma β stimulants should be given by oxygen driven nebuliser

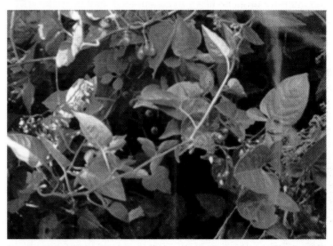

Atropa belladonna (deadly nightshade) contains several anticholinergic substances. Photo: Science U.com

Drug interactions with theophylline

	Effect
Increase in theophylline concentration	
Alcohol	Decreases theophylline clearance
Allopurinol	Decreased clearance
Cimetidine	Inhibits cytochrome P450, reducing clearance
Ciprofloxacin	As cimetidine
Interferon alfa	Marked decrease in clearance
Macrolides (erythromycin)	Decreased clearance
Oestrogen	Decreased clearance
Ticlopidine	Decreased clearance, concentrations may rise by 60%
Zafirlukast	Decreased clearance
Decrease in theophylline concentration	
Carbamazepine	50% increase in clearance
Cigarette smoking	Increased clearance around 30%
Phenytoin	Up to 70% increased clearance
Rifampicin	Increases cytochrome P450, increasing theophylline clearance up to 80%
Effect on other drugs	
Benzodiazepines	Larger doses of benzodiazepine may be required, effects may increase if theophylline is discontinued
Lithium	Lithium clearance increased
Pancuronium	Antagonised by theophylline, larger doses may be necessary

than 24 hours then blood concentrations should be measured and the rate adjusted as necessary.

Corticosteroids

Corticosteroids are effective in preventing the development of acute asthma.

Oral delivery

Oral prednisolone should be given if control of asthma is deteriorating despite usual regular treatment. A single oral dose of prednisolone, 40-50 mg according to body weight, should be given each day for at least five days until recovery, according to the speed of the response. If this opportunity is missed and an acute attack of asthma does develop corticosteroids are still an important element in treatment. No noticeable response occurs for four to six hours, so corticosteroids should be started as early as possible and intensive bronchodilator treatment used until they take effect.

Intravenous delivery

In most cases treatment with oral corticosteroids is adequate, but when there are life threatening features intravenous hydrocortisone should be used at an initial dose of 100 mg followed by 100 mg six hourly for 24 hours. Prednisolone should be started at a dose of 40-50 mg daily, whether or not hydrocortisone is used (50 mg prednisolone is equivalent to 200 mg hydrocortisone). If the patient is seen at home and then transferred to hospital the first dose of corticosteroid should be given together with initial bronchodilator treatment before the patient leaves home.

Length of steroid course

When intensive initial treatment has been required prednisolone should be maintained at 40 mg a day for at least a week. Two to three weeks of treatment may be needed to obtain the maximal response with deflation to normal lung volumes and loss of excessive diurnal variations of peak flow. Few side effects occur from such short courses of corticosteroids, but the most common ones are given in the adjacent box.

Steroids can be stopped abruptly after courses lasting up to three weeks. Tailing off the dose is not needed to prevent adrenal suppression or helpful to prevent relapse, although many patients are used to such regimens.

Oxygen

Acute severe asthma is always associated with hypoxia, though cyanosis develops late and is a grave sign. Death in asthma is caused by severe hypoxia; oxygen should be given as soon as possible. It is unusual to provoke carbon dioxide retention with oxygen treatment in asthma, so oxygen should be given freely during transfer to hospital where blood gas measurement can be made. Masks can provide 40-50% oxygen.

Nebulisers should be driven by oxygen whenever possible. In older people with an exacerbation of COPD there is a potential danger of carbon dioxide retention. In these patients treatment should begin with 24% or 28% oxygen by venturi mask until the results of blood gas measurements are available.

Magnesium

Intravenous magnesium sulphate is effective and safe in acute asthma. It is given as an infusion at a dose of 1.2-2.0 g over 20 minutes. It provides a possible additional therapy in acute severe asthma in hospital when the initial response to nebulised bronchodilators is inadequate.

Adverse effects of short course of oral corticosteroids
- Fluid retention
- Hyperglycaemia
- Indigestion
- Sleep disturbance
- Steroid induced psychosis
- Susceptibility to severe herpes zoster
- Weight gain

> Fatal attacks of asthma are associated with failure to prescribe any or adequate doses of corticosteroids

---

Side effects of short courses of corticosteroids
- Increased appetite
- Fluid retention
- Gastrointestinal upset
- Psychological disturbance

Exposure to herpes zoster may produce severe infections in susceptible individuals

---

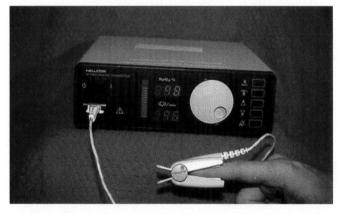

Supplemental oxygen is a very important component of the treatment of acute asthma. From Colquhoun M, et al (eds) *ABC of Resuscitation* 5th ed, Blackwell Publishing, 2004

> Studies have shown that nebulised isotonic magnesium sulphate adds to the bronchodilator effect of nebulised salbutamol

Fluid and electrolytes

Patients with acute asthma tend to be dehydrated because they are often too breathless to drink and because fluid loss from the respiratory tract is increased. Dehydration increases the viscosity of mucus, making plugging of the airways more likely, so intravenous fluid replacement is often necessary. Three litres should be given during the first 24 hours if little oral fluid is being taken.

Potassium supplements

Increased alveolar ventilation, sympathomimetic drugs, and corticosteroids all tend to lower the serum potassium concentration. This is the most common disturbance of electrolytes in acute asthma; the serum potassium concentration should be monitored and supplements given as necessary.

Antibiotics

Upper respiratory tract infections are the most common trigger factors for acute asthma and most of these are viral. In only a few cases are exacerbations of asthma precipitated by bacterial infection.

There is no evidence of benefit from the routine use of antibiotics. They should be reserved for patients in whom there is presumptive evidence of infection—such as fever, neutrophils in the blood or sputum, or radiological changes. Although all these features may occur in acute attacks without bacterial infection, an antibiotic such as amoxycillin, doxycycline, or erythromycin would be appropriate.

Controlled ventilation

Patients with acute severe asthma who need hospital admission should be treated in an area able to deal with acute medical emergencies, with adequate nursing and medical supervision. If hypoxia is worsening, hypercapnia is present, or patients are exhausted or drowsy, then they should be nursed in an intensive care unit.

Occasionally, mechanical ventilation may be necessary for a short time while the treatment takes effect. It is usually needed because the patient becomes exhausted; experience and careful observation are necessary to judge the right time to begin ventilatory support. Unlike in patients with COPD and restrictive lung disease, non-invasive ventilation is not usually appropriate in acute asthma, though it may occasionally be tried in expert hands in an intensive care unit.

High inflation pressures and long expiratory times may make ventilation difficult, but most experienced units have good results provided that the decision to ventilate the patient is made electively and is not precipitated by respiratory arrest. When patients being mechanically ventilated fail to improve on adequate treatment, bronchial lavage may occasionally be considered to reopen airways that have become plugged by mucus. In extremely severe unresponsive cases other treatments such as inhalational anaesthetics may be helpful, or a mixture of helium and oxygen may improve airflow while other treatment takes effect.

Other factors

Most patients with acute severe asthma improve with these measures. Occasionally physiotherapy may be useful to help patients cough up thick plugs of sputum, but mucolytic agents to change the nature of the secretions do not help.

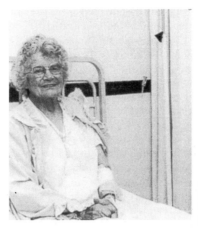

Some patients admitted to hospital with an acute attack will need intravenous rehydration

Immediate treatment	Life threatening features
Oxygen 40-60% Salbutamol 5 mg or terbutaline and ipratropium 0.5 mg by oxygen driven nebuliser Prednisolone 40-50 mg orally or hydrocortisone 100 mg intravenously No sedation Chest radiograph fairly soon	• Peak flow <33% predicted or best • Silent chest, feeble respiratory effort • Cyanosis, SaO$_2$ <92% • Bradycardia, hypotension, dysrhythmia • Exhaustion, confusion, coma • PCO$_2$ ≥4.6 kPa, PO$_2$ ≤8 kPa, acidosis

If life threatening features are present
• Discuss with ICU team
• IV magnesium sulphate 1.2-2 g iv over 20 minutes
• Frequent or continuous β$_2$ agonist nebulisation

Improving	Not improving after 15-30 minutes
Continue Oxygen Prednisolone 40-50 mg daily β agonist at least four hourly	Continue Oxygen and steroids β agonist up to every 15 minutes or continuously Ipratropium bromide 0.5 mg 4-6 hourly

Monitor	If still not improving
• Peak flow before and after nebulisations • Oximetry (keep saturation >92%) • Blood gas tensions if initial PaO$_2$ <8 kPa and saturation <93% *or* PaCO$_2$ normal or high *or* patient deteriorates	Aminophylline infusion 0.5 mg/kg/hour (monitor concentrations if longer than 24 hours) *or* Salbutamol or terbutaline infusion 5 to 15 μg/min

Treatment of acute severe asthma in hospital. Adapted from guidelines from the British Thoracic Society and Scottish Intercollegiate Guidelines Network

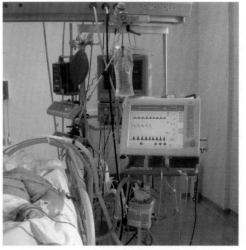

Mechanical ventilation is sometimes necessary in acute severe asthma

An episode of asthma is frightening. The dangerous use of sedatives such as morphine was common before effective treatment became available. Unfortunately this practice still continues, with occasional fatal consequences. Treatment of agitation should be aimed at reversing the asthma precipitating it, not at producing respiratory depression.

Discharge from hospital

Discharge too early is associated with increased readmission and mortality. Patients should have stopped nebuliser treatment and be using their own inhalers, with the proper technique checked, for at least 24 hours before discharge. Ideally peak flow should be above 75% of the patient's predicted or best known reading. Diurnal variability should be below 25%. A few patients may never lose their morning dips and may have to be discharged with them still present.

For every patient the reason for the acute episode should be sought and appropriate changes made in their routine treatment and in their response to any deterioration in an attempt to avoid similar attacks in the future. Patients with an acute attack of asthma should be looked after or at least seen by a physician with an interest in respiratory disease during their inpatient stay. Follow-up should be arranged, and a respiratory specialist nurse will be helpful in education, management, and support.

Subsequent management

At the time of their discharge patients should be stable on the treatment that they will take at home. They should leave with a plan of further management, which should include advice on asthma symptoms and peak flow measurement and a plan to respond to deterioration in the control of their asthma. The general practitioner should be informed of the admission and the subsequent plans and should see the patient within a week.

Hospital follow-up

The patient should return to the chest clinic within a month. Good communication between the hospital and the general practitioner is vital around this vulnerable period; and telephone, fax, and electronic links may help.

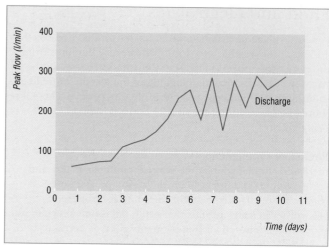

Peak flow during recovery from acute attack

Further reading

- Hughes R, Goldkorn A, Masoli M, Weatherall M, Burgess C, Beasley R. Use of isotonic nebulised magnesium sulphate as an adjuvant to salbutamol in treatment of severe asthma in adults: randomised placebo-controlled trial. *Lancet* 2003;361:2114-7.
- Silverman RA, Osborn H, Runge J, Gallagher EJ, Chiang W, Feldman J, et al. Acute Asthma/Magnesium Study Group. IV magnesium sulfate in the treatment of acute severe asthma: a multicenter randomized controlled trial. *Chest* 2002;122:489-97.

8 General management of chronic asthma

Guidelines

Various guidelines have been produced and published for the management of asthma. In the UK those produced by the British Thoracic Society and the Scottish Intercollegiate Guidelines Network, Asthma UK, and the Royal College of Physicians in association with accident and emergency, primary care, and paediatric groups have had wide distribution and acceptance. They were published in 2003 and updated in 2004. The Global Initiative for Asthma (GINA, www.ginasthma.com) also produces valuable guidelines and resources.

Guidelines are most likely to influence behaviour when they are adapted to local needs in hospital or practice and endorsed by a local respected enthusiast. They should be accompanied by regular audit against the agreed parts of the guidelines. Most of the published guidelines are in broad agreement on the strategy for managing chronic asthma.

In the UK the general practitioner contract allows practices to earn points related to organisation of asthma management.

General features

As a preliminary step in all patients with asthma, obvious precipitating factors should be sought and avoided when practicable. This is possible for specific allergens such as animals and foods but more difficult with widespread allergens such as pollens and house dust mites. A common non-specific stimulus is cigarette smoking. Up to a fifth of asthmatics continue to smoke; strenuous efforts should be made to discourage smoking in them and their families. Precipitating factors should be carefully explored on one of the first visits, but they should also be reassessed periodically.

Patients with asthma often look for a cure. It is important to establish early on that cure is not possible but if patients accept the need for regular treatment most can be virtually free from symptoms. Fortunately, most patients can achieve such control with safe drug treatment, with minimal or no side effects. Unfortunately, however, many patients with mild asthma fail to achieve this. Education in understanding the disease and treatment is often helped by home peak flow recording and written explanations of the purpose and practical details of treatment. In particular, the differences between symptomatic bronchodilator treatment and regular maintenance treatment must be emphasised. It is all too common to find asthmatic patients using their dose of inhaled steroid only to treat an acute attack. In general practice and in hospital, nurses provide a vital element in the management of asthma.

Inhaler technique and understanding of and adherence to management plans should be checked regularly, particularly when control is not adequate and stepping up treatment is being considered.

Asthma clinics

Many hospitals have concentrated their patients into specific asthma clinics for some years. Many general practices have specific asthma or respiratory disease clinics run by practice nurses. Others use the nurses in clinics for other chronic

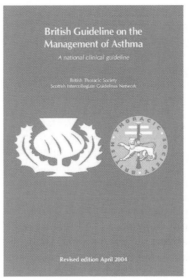

The BTS/SIGN guidelines are an excellent resource

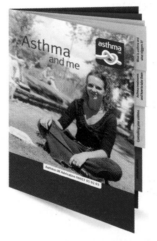
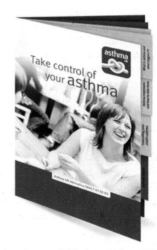

Some of the information for people with asthma available from Asthma UK (available through their website www.asthma.org.uk)

Levels of UK general practitioner contract related to asthma

- **Asthma 1** [7 points]—Register of patients with asthma receiving drugs in the past 12 months
- **Asthma 2** [15 points]—Diagnosis confirmed by spirometry or peak flow in up to 70% of patients aged >8 years diagnosed with asthma
- **Asthma 3** [6 points]—Record of smoking status in past 15 months in up to 70% of patients with asthma aged 14–19 years
- **Asthma 4** [6 points]—Record of smoking status in past 15 months in up to 70% of patients with asthma aged >20 years, except in those who have never smoked
- **Asthma 5** [6 points]—Record in notes that smoking cessation advice has been offered in past 15 months in up to 70% of patients with asthma who smoke
- **Asthma 6** [20 points]—Up to 70% of patients with asthma have been reviewed in previous 15 months
- **Asthma 7** [12 points]—Up to 70% of patients with asthma aged >16 years had influenza immunisation in preceding 1 September to 31 March

---

conditions as well as asthma. Local and national training courses are available for nurses who take on such clinics—for example, the National Respiratory Training Centre in Warwick. The clinics can be used to audit the treatment of asthmatic patients in a practice and to ensure that all patients are encouraged to participate in their optimal management.

Asthma clinics in general practice are best if they work with clearly written management guidelines and care plans. In some practices they are run by doctors but in most cases they are run by nurses, who have more time to spend with each individual patient to go through inhaler techniques, understanding, and management plans. An interested doctor should be available for consultation, and a close liaison should be built up with chest physicians at the local hospital. Every patient should have a personal management plan and be reviewed at least once a year.

Aims of management

Persistent inflammation of the airways and increased bronchial reactivity have been recognised even in mild intermittent asthma. Drugs such as inhaled corticosteroids, which reduce bronchial hyperresponsiveness, symptoms, and inflammatory infiltration of the airway, can target the inflammation. There has been a general move to more aggressive treatment of asthma, the goal being freedom from symptoms rather than tolerance of shortness of breath and frequent need of bronchodilators. Once control is achieved the regimen is usually maintained for three to six months before the treatment is stepped down.

Drug regimens
Routine regular use of short acting bronchodilators should be avoided. They should be used to treat symptoms, and their use should be limited by the use of prophylactic agents. This approach fits with the various sets of guidelines published over the past few years.

Regular inhaled corticosteroids decrease reactivity, as do leukotriene receptor antagonists and (probably) sodium cromoglicate and nedocromil sodium. Studies of mild asthma show that regular use of prophylactic agents reduces inflammation of the airways. The hope is that the reduction in the inflammation will prevent damage to the airway that would otherwise go on to produce irreversible obstruction. There is still no convincing long term evidence for this, nor is there convincing evidence that inhaled steroids change the natural course of asthma in any other way. Reactivity is improved but does not return to normal and reverts to pre-treatment levels when steroids are stopped. Leukotriene receptor antagonists have shown evidence of an anti-inflammatory action in addition to bronchodilatation.

Mild episodes of wheezing occurring once or twice a month can be controlled with inhaled β_2 agonists. When attacks are more frequent regular treatment with anti-inflammatory agent is necessary. Patients with lack of adequate control should be asked about sensitivity to irritants such as dust and smoke, night time symptoms, and peak flow recording. Definite diurnal variation on peak flow readings or nocturnal waking indicates a high degree of reactivity of the airways and the need for vigorous treatment. When chronic symptoms persist in the face of appropriate inhaled treatment a short course of oral corticosteroids often produces improvement, which may last for many months after the course.

Long acting inhaled β_2 agonists are good at controlling symptoms. They do not have a significant effect on underlying inflammation and should only be used in combination with inhaled steroids.

Control of asthma
The *British Guideline on the Management of Asthma* was first produced by the British Thoracic Society (BTS) and Scottish Intercollegiate Guidelines Network (SIGN) in January 2003 and updates have appeared since (www.sign.ac.uk/guidelines/fulltext/63/index.html).

The guidelines suggest that control of asthma should be assessed against the following standards:
- Minimal symptoms during day and night
- Minimal need for reliever medication
- No exacerbations
- Normal lung function (in practice FEV_1 and/or PEF $>80\%$ predicted or best)

This degree of control would be the aim for the first three steps in the guideline.

At steps four to five such freedom from symptoms may not be achievable without side effects, and the objectives are:
- Fewest possible symptoms
- Least possible need for relief bronchodilators
- Least possible limitation of activity
- Least possible PEF variation
- Best PEF
- Fewest adverse effects of treatment

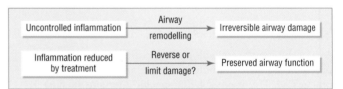

Aims of management of asthma

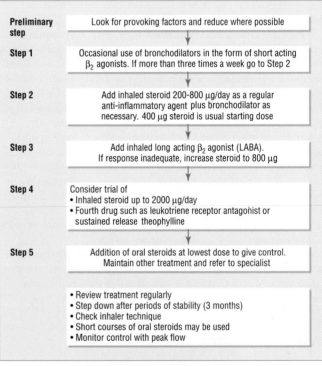

Stepwise treatment of asthma. Adapted from guidelines from the British Thoracic Society and Scottish Intercollegiate Guidelines Network.
The inhaled steroid would be beclometasone dipropionate, budesonide, or fluticasone propionate (starting at half the dose shown)

In a variable disease such as asthma, in which monitoring of the state of the disease is comparatively easy, the education and cooperation of the patient are vital parts of management. The patient should know how and when to take each treatment, broadly what each does, and exactly what to do in an exacerbation. These should be set out in a written plan specific for the individual patient.

Further reading

- British guideline on the management of asthma. www.brit-thoracic.org.uk/docs/asthmafull.pdf
- GINA Workshop Report, Global Strategy for Asthma Management and Prevention—updated 2004. Scientific information and recommendations for asthma programs. NIH Publication No. 02-3659. www.ginasthma.org

9 Treatment of chronic asthma

β agonists

The first line of treatment for the relief of asthma is one of the selective β_2 agonists taken by inhalation. β_2 agonists are the most effective bronchodilator in asthma. They start to work quickly—salbutamol and terbutaline take effect within 15 minutes and last for four to six hours. There is no clear threshold for all patients, but if there has been an exacerbation of asthma in the past two years, if inhaled β_2 agonists are needed three times a week or more, or if symptoms are present three times a week or waking one night a week, then additional treatment must be considered. The dose response varies among patients as does the dose that will produce side effects, such as tremor. Patients should be taught to monitor their inhaler use and to understand that if they need it more, or if its effects lessen, these are danger signals. They indicate deterioration in control and the need for further treatment.

Adverse effects

Some patients worry that β_2 agonists may become slightly less effective with time, particularly if the dose is high. There is little evidence of appreciable tachyphylaxis for the airway effects in asthmatics. If it exists, it is minor and is quickly reversed by stopping the treatment temporarily or by taking corticosteroids. Tremor, palpitations, and muscle cramps may occur but are rarely troublesome if the drug is inhaled; these adverse effects often become less of a problem with continued treatment.

Some studies found that regular use of β_2 agonists was associated with increased bronchial reactivity, worsening control of asthma, and accelerated decline of lung function. These have not been confirmed, and when the standard guidelines are followed, β_2 agonists are not used regularly unless they are needed for control of symptoms.

Long acting β agonists

The long acting inhaled β_2 agonists salmeterol and formoterol have had an increasing role in treatment since the early 1990s. The mechanism of the prolonged action is different in the two drugs and the onset of bronchodilatation is faster with formoterol, but in other ways most physicians regard them as equivalent. Choice depends more on the device required than the drug itself. They are particularly effective for nocturnal and exercise induced asthma. The British guidelines now place them as a first option at "step 3," when a low to moderate dose of inhaled corticosteroids (400-800 µg beclometasone or equivalent) fails to establish symptom-free control.

Several studies have shown that salmeterol and formoterol are is more effective than doubling the intake of inhaled corticosteroids in controlling symptoms and increasing peak flow. The effect is maintained over six months in such studies. A comparison of low and high dose inhaled steroids over 12 months, with or without formoterol, showed that increasing steroids and addition of formoterol reduced exacerbations. Severe exacerbations, defined by the need for oral steroids or peak flow drop, were prevented more effectively by higher dose steroids than formoterol, but best of all by the combination. Formoterol with steroids was the most effective in symptom reduction and peak flow control. Remember, long acting β agonists are bronchodilators and do not suppress inflammation.

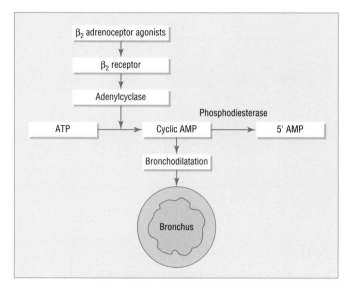

Increases in cyclic AMP lead to bronchodilatation and may be produced by β_2 receptor stimulation or phosphodiesterase inhibition

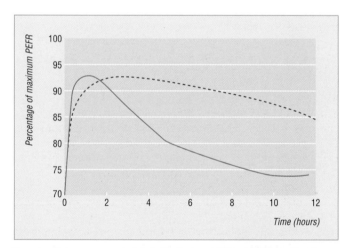

Bronchodilator response to inhaled salbutamol 200 µg (solid line) and inhaled salmeterol 50 µg (broken line). Adapted from Ullman A et al, *Thorax* 1988;43:674-8

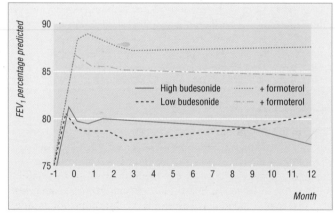

Effect of formoterol with and without a corticosteroid. Adapted from Pauwels RA et al, *N Engl J Med* 1997;337:1405-11

In asthma they should always be given with inhaled steroids, and the patient must not stop taking these on finding a highly effective medication. In addition they should carry a short acting β agonist to use for acute symptoms. Adverse effects of salmeterol and formoterol are the same as those of short acting agents.

Anticholinergic bronchodilators

Ipratropium bromide blocks the cholinergic bronchoconstrictor effect of the vagus nerve. It is a non-selective antagonist blocking inhibitory M1 receptors on postganglionic nerves as well as M3 receptors on airway smooth muscle. A longer acting agent—tiotropium—is available for COPD.

Effectiveness
Anticholinergics are most effective in very young children and in older patients. They are as effective or more effective than β_2 agonists in COPD. In asthma, anticholinergic agents are less effective than β_2 agonists, but they may supplement their effect if reversibility is incomplete. They may be useful in patients with troublesome tremor or tachycardia.

Methylxanthines

Theophylline is an effective bronchodilator and may also have some anti-inflammatory actions. Its safety margin is lower than other inhalational bronchodilators. Individual differences in the doses required are high so it is necessary to monitor treatment by blood concentrations. Inhaled treatment with β agonists is preferable, but slow release theophyllines are an alternative to long acting β agonists for nocturnal symptoms. Absorption of aminophylline from suppositories is much less predictable, and they are best avoided.

Adverse effects
The starting dose of theophylline should be around 7 mg/kg/day in divided doses and should then be built up. All patients taking theophylline should have their serum concentrations monitored and doses adjusted until they are between 8 and 18 mg/l (40-90 μmol/l) for optimal bronchodilator effect. Above 20 mg/l toxic effects are unacceptably high, though gastrointestinal effects are common at lower concentrations.

Smoking, alcohol consumption, and enzyme-inducing drugs such as phenytoin, rifampicin, and barbiturates increase theophylline clearance (p.29). Clearance will be decreased and blood concentrations will rise if it is given at the same time as cimetidine, ciprofloxacin, or erythromycin and in patients with heart failure, liver impairment, or pneumonia.

Lower theophylline concentrations, with a lower risk of side effects, have an anti-inflammatory effect in vivo and in vitro. This is a possible alternative, at levels of 5-15 mg/l, at steps 2 and 3 but leukotriene receptor antagonists offer a better alternative to inhaled steroids where this is necessary.

Mast cell stabilisers

Sodium cromoglicate
Sodium cromoglicate blocks bronchoconstrictor responses to challenge by exercise and antigens. The original proposed mechanism of stabilisation of mast cells may not be the main mechanism of its action in asthma. Sodium cromoglicate is less effective than inhaled corticosteroids. With the introduction of leukotriene receptor antagonists there is little reason to prescribe cromoglicate.

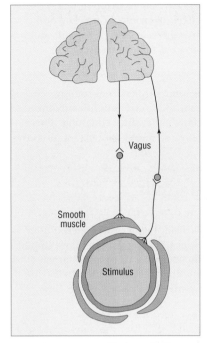

Anticholinergic agents block vagal efferent stimulation of bronchial smooth muscle

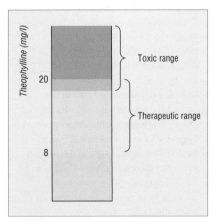

There is no safety margin between therapeutic and toxic ranges with theophylline

Side effects of theophylline

Most common are:
- Nausea
- Vomiting
- Abdominal discomfort

However, the following side effects can occur, sometimes without early warning from gastrointestinal symptoms
- Headache
- Malaise
- Fast pulse rate
- Fits

Other mast cell stabilisers have been disappointing, possibly because of the additional effects of cromoglicate. The oral agent ketotifen produces drowsiness in 10% of patients and has little activity, although it is used in some countries.

Nedocromil sodium
Nedocromil sodium has the same properties as sodium cromoglicate but may have an additional anti-inflammatory effect on the airway epithelium and reduce coughing. There is still little reason to use it, however, unless patients will not take inhaled steroids.

Inhaled corticosteroids

Inhaled corticosteroids are the most effective preventative treatment in asthma. Steroids may be given by metered dose inhaler, dry powder devices, or nebuliser, and the dose should be adjusted to give optimum control. Two common inhaled steroids—beclometasone dipropionate and budesonide—are roughly equivalent in dose, while fluticasone has the same effect at half the dose.

Method of delivery
The formulation and delivery device must also be considered. The non-CFC beclometasone metered dose inhaler QVar has a small particle size and increased lung deposition. The dose of beclometasone can be halved when the patient is switched from another preparation. Much of the benefit of inhaled corticosteroids is seen at low to moderate doses up to 400-800 µg beclometasone. There is some further effect with higher doses but the dose response above 800 µg beclometasone or 500 µg fluticasone becomes flatter.

Adverse effects
In adults there are no problems, apart from occasional oropharyngeal candidiasis or a husky voice, until a daily dose above the equivalent of 1000 µg beclometasone dipropionate is reached. At higher doses there may be biochemical evidence of suppression of the hypothalamic-pituitary-adrenal axis, even with inhaled steroids. Much of the systemic effect comes from absorption from the lung itself, bypassing the metabolic pathways of the gut and liver that limit any problems from drug deposited in the mouth and swallowed.

With doses of more than 1000 µg daily of budesonide or beclometasone there are metabolic effects, including an increase in the concentration of osteocalcin, a marker of increased bone turnover. There is some evidence of skin thinning and purpura, even in patients who have not had appreciable doses of oral steroids. Doses over 2000 µg daily are not often used, but when necessary nebulised budesonide or fluticasone may be a convenient strategy. At doses of >800 µg daily a large volume spacer should be used to reduce pharyngeal deposition associated with metered dose inhalers. At ≥1000 µg it is advisable for patients to carry a steroid card, especially if they use occasional courses of oral steroids.

Regular use
Doses of inhaled steroids should be taken regularly to be effective. Twice daily use is the usual frequency. In milder asthma under good control once daily use may be adequate. Doubling the regular dose when an upper respiratory infection develops is not beneficial.

Adherence
The main difficulties in the use of inhaled corticosteroids are the patients' worries about the use of steroids and the difficulties

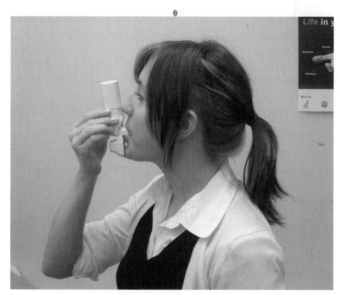
The Autoinhaler is triggered by inspiratory airflow. Breath actuated metered dose inhalers are available for β agonists, anticholinergics, cromoglicate, and corticosteroids

---

Side effects of inhaled corticosteroids

Established	Suggested at high dose
• Oropharyngeal candidiasis	• Adrenal suppression
• Dysphonia	• Reduced growth in children
• Irritation and cough	• Osteoporosis
• Purpura and thinning of skin	
• Cataracts	

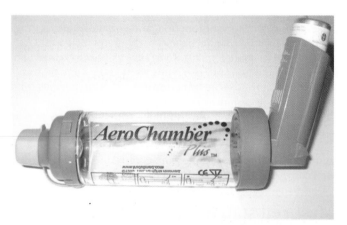
Large volume spacers overcome problems with coordination of inhaler firing and inspiration. They reduce oropharyngeal deposition of the aerosol and improve delivery to the lungs. A smaller volume spacer such as the one above is more convenient and seems to be as efficient as larger volume chambers. With permission from GlaxoSmithKline

of ensuring that they take regular medication even when they are well. These problems may be increased by the use of inhaled corticosteroids earlier in the course of asthma and to achieve total control free of symptoms. Combination with long acting bronchodilators may improve adherence as loss of bronchodilator effect will be noticed more quickly if therapy is discontinued.

Dosage reduction

There seems to be no advantage in starting a high dose to achieve quicker control. The starting dose should match the severity of the asthma, and moderate doses are usually adequate and appropriate. When asthma is controlled the next decision is how long to maintain the inhaled steroids. The dose should be reviewed regularly, particularly at doses >1000 µg daily. Control should be established for three months before the dose is reduced by 25-50%, though more flexible regimens to match the dose to symptoms are also used.

Oral corticosteroids

Short courses of oral steroids are often necessary for acute exacerbations and have few serious problems. Some patients have to take long term oral corticosteroids but this should be only after vigorous treatment with other drugs has failed. The symptoms or risks of the disease must be balanced against the adverse effects of long term treatment with oral corticosteroids.

Length of treatment

Short courses of oral steroids may be stopped abruptly or tailed off over a few days. Low concentrations of cortisol and adrenocorticotrophic hormone (ACTH) are found for just two to three days after 40 mg prednisolone daily for three weeks, but clinical problems with responses to stress or exacerbations of asthma do not occur. An appropriate course would be 30-50 mg prednisolone daily for a minimum of five days and usually up to 14 days until baseline function returns. Most patients can be taught to keep such a supply of steroids at home and to use them according to their individual management plan when predetermined signs of deteriorating control occur.

If patients require long term oral steroids, they should be settled on a regimen of treatment on alternate days whenever possible. The goal is always to establish control with other treatments so that the oral steroids can be discontinued. Inhaled steroids in moderate to high doses should be maintained to keep the oral dose as low as possible. Alternative preparations such as ACTH and triamcinolone are less flexible and give no appreciable benefit in terms of adrenal suppression.

Adverse effects

When patients are on long term oral steroids or take short courses more than three times a year the risks of osteoporosis should be considered. Patients at high risk—such as those aged ≥65—should start taking protective treatment when they start regular steroids. Regular exercise and adequate dietary vitamin D and calcium intake should be encouraged in all patients on oral steroids. Patients on steroids should be advised to avoid contact with chickenpox and herpes zoster while they are taking the drugs and for three months after prolonged use. Blood glucose concentrations and blood pressure should be monitored in patients on regular oral steroids.

Leukotriene antagonists

The leukotriene receptor antagonists are the first wholly new class of drugs to have become available for asthma in the past 20 years. The cysteinyl leukotrienes LTC4, LTD4, and LTE4 are

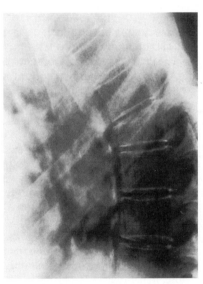

Deposition of beclometasone dipropionate after use of CRF containing metered dose inhaler and the CFC free Qvar inhaler (from Leach CL, *Respir Med* 1998;92(suppl A0:3-8).The latter produces a substantial increase in lung deposition (3M Healthcare)

> **Resistance—A few asthmatic patients are fully or partially resistant to corticosteroids. They form a particularly difficult group to treat**

Osteoporotic collapse of a thoracic vertebra in a patient taking oral steroids

> **Advice can be found at the National Osteoporosis Society website** www.nos.org.uk/glucocorticoid.asp

inflammatory mediators formed from arachidonic acid by the action of the enzyme 5-lipoxygenase. These leukotrienes produce bronchoconstriction, oedema, mucus secretion, eosinophil recruitment, and inflammation in the airway. Drugs such as montelukast and zafirlukast act as competitive inhibitors of receptors on smooth muscle and elsewhere. The other potential target is inhibition of 5-lipoxygenase itself.

Leukotriene receptor antagonists are available only for oral use. They should be taken an hour or two before or after food. Side effects are rare. They have been associated with Churg-Strauss syndrome (allergic granulomatosis) but this is usually unmasking of the underlying problem by the reduction in steroid treatment possible after addition of zafirlukast.

Leukotriene receptor antagonists have been used in various settings: as alternatives to inhaled steroids in prevention, as an alternative to long acting β agonists, and as an additional treatment when control is difficult. Overall the effects seem to be less than those achieved with inhaled steroids, and they should be regarded as second choice to inhaled steroids for patients needing more than occasional short acting bronchodilators. Nevertheless, they may be useful in patients who are not prepared to take inhaled steroids or have adverse responses or in those with exercise or aspirin induced asthma.

These agents have an action as an add on therapy to inhaled steroids. However, more evidence exists to support the use of long acting β agonists and these remain the treatment of choice in patients not controlled on low to moderate dose inhaled steroids. There is evidence that leukotriene receptor antagonists can reduce exacerbations and allow reduction in inhaled steroid dose when used as additional therapy. Overall they are a useful adjunct to the treatment and have the benefit of an effect on associated rhinitis.

Steroid sparing agents

In patients requiring oral steroids to maintain control, several other agents have been used to try to reduce the steroid dose and avoid the associated side effects. All these treatments have side effects of their own and should be used under specialist advice with all other conventional treatments in place.

Methotrexate—There have been several trials of methotrexate, usually taken orally once a week. Around half of these have had positive results, with a significant reduction in steroid dose, and a trial of two to three months' treatment may be appropriate in some patients. Adverse effects are on bone marrow, liver, and lungs.

Other agents—Ciclosporin and oral gold have been effective in some studies, producing some improvement in control with a small decrease in steroid dose. Renal toxicity is a problem with both agents.

Desensitisation and avoidance of allergens

As discussed in chapter 5, the results of trials of desensitisation and avoidance of allergens have produced limited benefit. Some patients have obvious precipitating factors—in particular animals—and avoidance is helpful, but there are usually other unknown precipitating factors. More common are patients with reactive airways who are also sensitive to pollens, house dust mite, and other allergens. Such stimuli are almost impossible to avoid completely in everyday life, though symptoms can improve with rigorous measures. It is sensible to try to reduce the exposure to known allergens as much as possible.

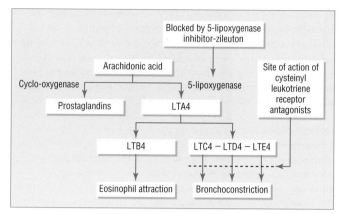

Site of action of drugs affecting the leukotriene system

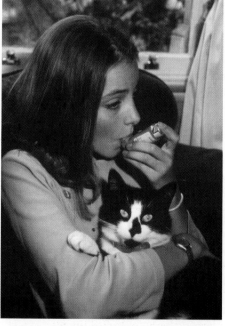

Leukotriene receptor agonists may be useful for those with exercise induced asthma

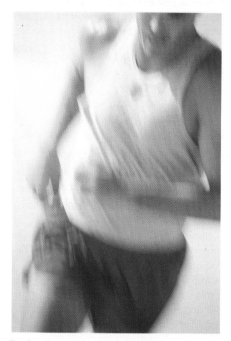

Avoiding contact with animals can be helpful for some patients with asthma. With permission of Mark Clarke/Science Photo Library

In children at risk of asthma it may be particularly important to limit their exposure to potential allergic triggers.

There is some evidence that desensitisation is beneficial in patients with asthma who are sensitive to pollens and that repeated courses increase the improvement. Several studies of house mite desensitisation in children have suggested some benefit, but these were highly selected groups; it is unusual to find asthmatic patients with a single sensitivity. The degree of control produced by desensitisation can usually be achieved with simple, safe, inhaled drugs.

Newer techniques such as peptide immunotherapy raise the possibility of more effective and safer treatment using higher doses of modified antigen.

There is little sound evidence to support desensitisation to other agents in asthmatic patients. In particular, cocktails produced from the results of skin or radioallergosorbent tests are not a valid form of treatment. Local reactions to desensitising agents are common and more generalised reactions and even death can occur. Most deaths have been related to errors in the injection schedule and inadequate supervision after injections. Desensitisation should be undertaken only where appropriate facilities for resuscitation are available.

Combined preparations

Some fixed dose combinations are available for the treatment of asthma. Combinations of bronchodilators may be used when each component has been shown to be appropriate at the dose in the fixed combination. This is unusual in asthma.

Combinations of long acting inhaled bronchodilators and corticosteroids are convenient in many patients and may improve adherence. Combinations of formoterol and budesonide can be varied with the severity and symptoms as both budesonide and formoterol doses can be varied over a reasonable range. Salmeterol is usually restricted to a dose of 50 mg twice daily. Combined preparations of salmeterol and fluticasone are used to attain more prolonged periods of complete asthma control before adjustment of the dose rather than more frequent adjustments in response to symptoms, which has been used successfully with the formoterol budesonide combination.

Alternative treatments

Many asthmatic patients turn to alternative therapies in the management of their asthma. Most will use these alongside conventional treatment but may not inform their medical carers, particularly if they appear dismissive of such treatments. The dangers come when alternative treatments are used instead of standard treatments. Controlled trials are more difficult in this area, and there are few examples of scientifically valid trials of adequate size and duration. Few of these techniques have been shown to have measurable benefit in scientifically rigorous studies. It is best to work with patients who want to try these techniques, however, by encouraging them to maintain conventional treatment alongside any other therapies.

Acupuncture—Control in trials is again often inadequate because the elements of treatment associated with the use of acupuncture needles make sham treatments difficult. Short term studies have shown some benefit, but these do not compare with those of conventional pharmacological treatment.

Relaxation, yoga, hypnotherapy—Various approaches have shown benefit in individual trials but none have been shown to be effective consistently in properly controlled studies. Hypnosis has been shown to have some effect, particularly in susceptible patients.

> **Other challenges**—One area where desensitisation is appropriate is in sensitivity to insect venom that results in anaphylaxis rather than asthma. Aspirin induced asthma may respond to careful oral desensitisation

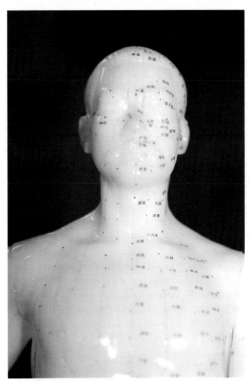

Acupuncture can be used to complement conventional therapy (photos.com)

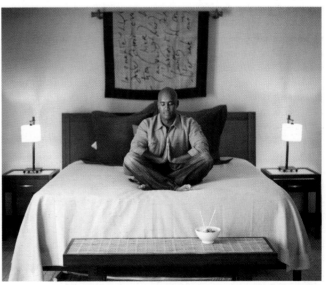

Yoga has been used by some patients to manage their asthma (photos.com)

Breathing exercises—The Buteyko technique of breathing control has been promoted as an effective treatment of asthma. One of the benefits may be to reduce respiratory rate and hyperventilation. There does seem to be a small benefit in symptoms and bronchodilator use in controlled studies.

Homoeopathy—There have been suggestions of improvement in some studies, either in symptoms without change in FEV_1 or small changes in lung function. However, there remains a lack of high quality studies.

Ionisation—Inspiration of ionised air may have a small effect on lung function and may attenuate the response to exercise, but such effects are limited and the degree of ionisation is not achieved by the widely advertised home ionisers. There is even some suggestion that these may make nocturnal cough worse, and there is no indication to use them.

Massage and spinal manipulation—These techniques have been popular but have not been shown to have any benefit in the few controlled studies.

Speleotherapy—Descent in to subterranean environments is a common approach in central and eastern Europe. Some studies have shown short term benefit, but adequate controlled trials are needed. Moving to high altitudes where there are low levels of pollution and allergen is a traditional approach with short term benefits but no evidence of a continued effect on return to the usual environment.

Traditional and herbal medicines—It is likely that some of these preparations contain potentially useful agents. There are difficulties in standardisation of products, however, and some have been found to contain agents such as corticosteroids with the usual side effects.

Future treatments

There are other exciting possibilities of drugs that affect the inflammatory pathway or modulate the immunological response. Monoclonal antibodies against IgE have been shown to be effective in asthma if IgE levels are reduced far enough. This is the first biotechnology therapy to be licensed for use in some countries. It has been shown to suppress early and late asthmatic reactions, reduce exacerbations, and improve symptoms scores and to be steroid sparing in severe asthma. Serum IgE levels need to be reduced by more than 95%. Other mediator antagonists are likely to follow on from the leukotriene receptor antagonists. Inhibition of Th2 cytokines such as anti-IL15 involved in eosinophil maturation and IL13 offer possibilities. Interference with Th1/Th2 balance might be possible but could have other immunological consequences. Other potential targets under study include antagonists of chemokines, adhesion molecules, tumour necrosis factor, and inhibitors of phosphodiesterase type 4 (PDE-4 inhibitors).

Inhibitors of tryptase (a serine protease released from mast cells) and nitric oxide production are other topics under active investigation. The range of such treatments will probably increase over the next few years.

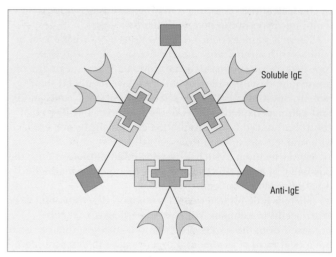

Anti-IgE binds to soluble IgE to form inactive hexamers and stop IgE cross linking and degranulating mast cells

Further reading

- Bateman ED, Boushey HA, Bousquet J, Busse WW, Clark TJ, Pauwels RA, et al. Can guideline-defined asthma control be achieved? The gaining optimal asthma control study. GOAL investigators group. *Am J Respir Crit Care Med* 2004;170:836-44.
- Cooper S, Oborne J, Newton S, Harrison V, Thompson Coon J, Lewis S, et al. Effect of two breathing exercises (Buteyko and pranayama) in asthma: a randomised controlled trial. *Thorax* 2003;58:674-9.
- Ducharme F, Schwartz Z, Hicks G, Kakuma R. Addition of anti-leukotriene agents to inhaled corticosteroids for chronic asthma. *Cochrane Database Syst Rev* 2004;(2):CD003133.
- Holt S, Suder A, Weatherall M, Cheng S, Shirtcliffe P, Beasley R. Dose-response of inhaled fluticasone propionate in adolescents and adults with asthma: meta-analysis. *BMJ* 2001;323:253-6.
- Ilowite J, Webb R, Friedman B, Kerwin E, Bird SR, Hustad CM, et al. Addition of montelukast or salmeterol to fluticasone for protection against asthma attacks: a randomized, double-blind, multicenter study. *Ann Allergy Asthma Immunol* 2004;92:641-8.
- Ind PW, Haughney J, Price D, Rosen JP, Kennelly J. Adjustable and fixed dosing with budesonide/formoterol via a single inhaler in asthma patients: the ASSURE study. *Respir Med* 2004;98:464-75.
- Leach CL. Improved delivery of inhaled steroids to the large and small airways. *Respir Med* 1998;92(suppl A):3-8.
- O'Byrne PM, Bisgaard H, Godard PP, Pistolesi M, Palmqvist M, Zhu Y, et al. Budesonide/formoterol combination therapy as both maintenance and reliever medication in asthma. *Am J Respir Crit Care Med* 2005;171:129-36.
- Pauwels RA, Lofdahl CG, Postma DS, Tattersfield AE, O'Byrne P, Barnes PJ, et al. Effect of inhaled formoterol and budesonide on exacerbations of asthma. Formoterol and corticosteroids establishing therapy (FACET) international study group. *N Engl J Med* 1997;337:1405-11.

10 Methods of delivering drugs

Various inhaler devices and formulations have been developed to deliver drugs efficiently, minimise side effects, and simplify use. With the range of devices available nearly all patients can take drugs by inhalation. All the available devices used appropriately can provide adequate drug to the airways. Inhalers should not be prescribed without checking that the patient can use the device satisfactorily. This should be rechecked on subsequent visits as errors can develop and interfere with treatment. Some drugs, such as leukotriene receptor antagonists and theophylline, cannot be given by inhalation.

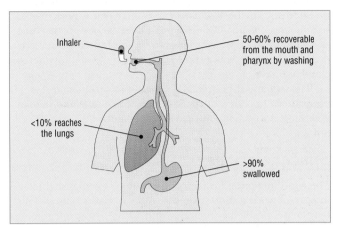
Inhalers deliver the drug direct to the airways

Metered dose inhalers

Inhalers deliver the drug directly to the airways. Even when a metered dose inhaler (MDI) is used properly, however, only about 10% of the drug reaches the airways below the larynx. Nearly all the rest of the drug gets no further than the oropharynx and is swallowed. This swallowed portion may be absorbed from the gastrointestinal tract, but drugs such as inhaled corticosteroids are largely removed by first pass metabolism in the liver. Absorption directly from the lung bypasses liver metabolism.

An MDI should be shaken and then fired into the mouth shortly after the start of a slow full inspiration. At full inflation the breath should be held for 10 seconds. The technique should be checked periodically. About a quarter of patients have difficulty using a metered dose inhaler and the problems increase with age. Arthritic patients can find it hard to activate the inhaler and may be helped by a Haleraid device, which responds to squeezing, or be given a breath actuated or dry powder system.

Breath actuated aerosol inhalers

Breath actuated MDIs are available for most classes of drug. The valve on the inhaler is actuated as the patient breathes in. The devices respond to a low inspiratory flow rate and are useful for those who have difficulty coordinating actuation and breathing. They require a propellant similar to that found in a standard inhaler.

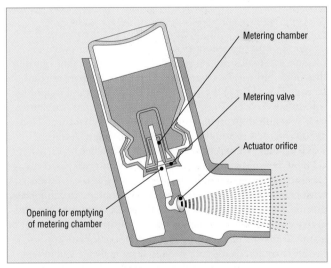
The mechanisms inside a metered dose inhaler

CFC-free inhalers

Many current MDIs have moved from chlorofluorocarbon (CFC) propellants. The production, importation, and use of CFCs have been stopped in most developed countries because of the effect on the ozone layer. There is a temporary exemption for medical use under the Montreal Protocol, but CFC inhalers will be removed once adequate non-CFC products become available.

Alternative propellants

The challenge has been to develop safe alternatives that are as convenient, effective, and clinically equivalent. The process of development of alternative propellants has been more of a problem than first appreciated, particularly for inhaled steroids. Adaptations to the method of adding the drug to the propellant and to the valve and jet mechanisms have been necessary.

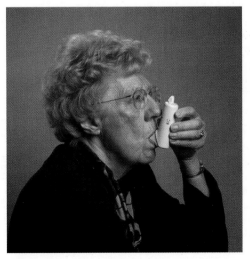
Elderly patients may find using a metered dose inhaler difficult (3M United Kingdom plc)

Hydrofluoroalkanes (HFAs) 134 and 227 are used in the new devices.

Short and long acting β agonists, inhaled steroids, and combinations are now available in inhalers with hydrofluoroalkanes. Each new device has to be tested carefully as total and regional delivery to the lung will differ with the new devices. The beclometasone product QVar is prescribed at half the dose of a conventional MDI because of its better lung deposition. Other preparations can be substituted at the same dose. Patients will notice differences in the speed of the aerosol cloud and taste.

The switch to CFC-free MDIs should be taken as an opportunity to review the patient's understanding and inhaler technique and general asthma management.

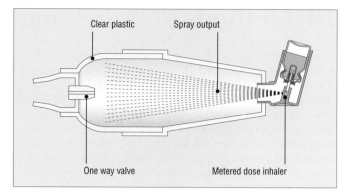

An extension tube (spacer) used with a metered dose inhaler. Some large volume spacers are being replaced by smaller volume devices

Spacer devices

The coordination of firing and inspiration becomes slightly less important when a short extension tube or spacer is used. This may help if problems are minor, and a larger reservoir removes the need for coordination of breathing and actuation. The inhaler is fixed into the chamber and the breath is taken through a one way valve at the other end of the chamber. Inhalation should be as soon as possible after each actuation, certainly within 30 seconds, and tidal breathing is as effective as deep breaths.

Pharyngeal deposition is greatly reduced as the faster particles strike the walls of the chamber, not the mouth. Evaporation of propellant from the larger, slower particles produces a small sized aerosol that penetrates further out into the lungs and deposits a greater proportion of drug beyond the larynx. This reduces the risk of oral candidiasis and dysphonia with inhaled corticosteroids and reduces potential problems with systemic absorption from the gastrointestinal tract. They should be used routinely when doses of inhaled steroid of >800 µg daily are given by metered dose inhaler.

The device is cumbersome, but this is no great disadvantage for twice daily treatment such as corticosteroids. Chambers have proved useful as a substitute for a nebuliser in acute asthma. Output characteristics of MDIs vary, and inhalers and extension tubes need to be matched appropriately. It cannot be assumed that results transfer to different combinations.

Electrostatic charge can reduce drug delivery. Chambers should be washed in detergent and left to air dry (rather than wiped dry) once a month and changed every 6–12 months. Metal chambers without static charge can also be used.

Use of spacer devices
- Match the MDI and spacer
- Inhale as soon as possible after each single actuation
- Empty the chamber by single large breaths or tidal breathing
- Clean chamber monthly
- Wash chamber in detergent and water and leave to dry
- Wipe any detergent from mouthpiece
- Replace spacer every 6-12 months

Dry powder inhalers

Dry powder inhalers of various types are available for β agonists, sodium cromoglicate, corticosteroids, anticholinergic agents, and combinations. Because inspiratory airflow releases the fine powder many problems of coordination are avoided, and there are none of the environmental worries of metered dose inhalers. The dry powder makes some patients cough, and the respiratory flow rate needed may be a problem with some devices in asthma. The problems of reloading for each dose have been eased by the development of multiple dose units with up to 200 doses and many devices have a dose counter that helps the patient to know when the inhaler needs renewing and provides a compliance monitor.

Some dry powder devices such as the Turbohaler increase lung deposition and may allow a reduction in the prescribed dose.

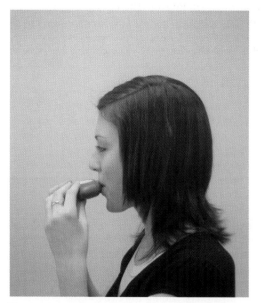

The Accuhaler has a convenient dose counter

Nebulisers

Nebulisers can be driven by compressed gas (jet nebuliser) or an ultrasonically vibrating crystal (ultrasonic nebuliser). They provide a way of giving inhaled drugs to those unable to use any other device—for example, the very young—or in acute attacks when inspiratory flow is limited.

Nebulisers also offer a convenient way of delivering a higher dose to the airways. Generally, about 12% of the drug leaving the chamber enters the lungs, but most of the dose stays in the apparatus or is wasted in expiration. Delivery depends on the type of nebuliser chamber, the flow rate at which it is driven, and the volume in the chamber. In most cases flow rates of less than 6 l/min in a jet nebuliser give too large a particle and nebulise too slowly. Some chambers have a reservoir and valve system to reduce loss to the surrounding room during expiration.

In many situations equivalent effects can be obtained with MDI and a spacer but patients often have confidence in their nebuliser.

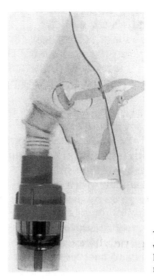

The use of nebulisers must be associated with careful instructions on use and hygiene as well as arrangements for maintenance and support

Tablets and syrups

Tablets and syrups are available for oral use. This route is necessary for theophyllines and leukotriene antagonists, which cannot be inhaled effectively. Very young children who are unable to inhale drugs can take the sugar-free liquid preparations. Slow release tablets are used when a prolonged action is needed, particularly for nocturnal asthma in which theophyllines have proved helpful. Various slow release mechanisms or long acting drugs have been developed to maintain even blood concentrations.

Tablets avoid the need to learn the coordination required for inhalers and might allow delivery to lung tissue beyond blocked airways but at the expense of potential side effects from body distribution.

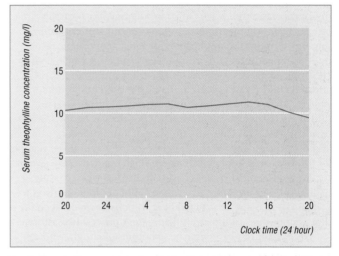

Steady theophylline concentrations in the therapeutic range can be obtained with twice daily slow release preparations (D'Alonzo GE et al, *Am Rev Respir Dis* 1990;142:84-90)

Injections and infusions

Injections are used for the treatment of acute attacks. Subcutaneous injections may be useful in emergencies when nebulisers are unavailable. Occasional patients with severe chronic asthma seem to benefit from the high levels of β stimulant obtained with subcutaneous infusion through a portable pump. Rates may need to be adjusted depending on severity. The infusion site is changed by the patient every one to three days.

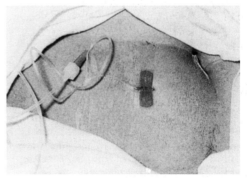

In severe case β₂ agonists can be delivered by subcutaneous infusion

ASTHMA IN CHILDREN – Dipak Kanabar

11 Definition, prevalence, and prevention

Defining asthma in children

Childhood asthma contains a spectrum of disorders that exhibit various clinical and pathological features. Labelling a child as asthmatic can still cause anxiety within the family and controversy among paediatricians. Alternative diagnoses such as wheezy bronchitis or allergic airways disease, however, probably hinder clinicians in their approach to management of asthma.

Presenting symptoms

For most practising paediatricians and general practitioners, a preschool child with recurrent wheezy episodes whose wheeze disappears after treatment with a bronchodilator probably justifies a clinical diagnosis of asthma (on the understanding that this term has no implication for long term prognosis or underlying pathology). For example, respiratory syncitial virus (RSV) bronchiolitis itself causes wheezing and up to half of affected children will go on to develop recurrent episodic wheeze. Many children have mild wheezing during viral infections (virus associated wheeze), but their prognosis is better than children who have wheeze without a viral infection. In addition, the airways of children in the first two to three years of life (that is, preschool children) are small relative to the size of the lungs. The airways and chest walls are less rigid, so during expiration they are more likely than those of older children to collapse or become obstructed by secretions or mucosal changes that are not the result of an inflammatory process like asthma.

Older children can describe symptoms of cough, wheeze, dyspnoea, and chest tightness, and whether there is an improvement with bronchodilator and steroid therapy. In addition, peak flow measurements, FEV_1 by spirometry, exercise testing, and recordings of diurnal variations will assist diagnosis.

Thus in paediatric practice, in the absence of an easily recognised diagnostic marker, a clinical diagnosis of asthma usually relies on a combination of history of characteristic symptoms, evidence of airway lability, and, in particular, a reduction in symptoms after treatment with a short acting β_2 agonist showing reversible airflow obstruction.

Prevalence of asthma

Asthma is the most common chronic disease of childhood. About 1 in 6 (17%) or more children aged between 2 and 15 in the UK have asthma symptoms that require treatment.

Is prevalence increasing or reaching a plateau?

While several epidemiological studies show that the prevalence of asthma and other atopic disorders such as eczema and hay fever is increasing in many countries throughout the world, more recent studies indicate that, perhaps in the Western world at least, prevalence rates are reaching a plateau.

The observation that all forms of allergic disease are increasing simultaneously suggests an increase in host susceptibility, rather than a rise in allergic sensitisation. Associations between the prevalence of asthma and small family size, affluence, and BCG status (decreased asthma with BCG vaccine) are all recognised and, coupled with our understanding

The International Consensus Report on the Diagnosis and Management of Asthma gives the following definition: "Asthma is a chronic inflammatory disorder of the airway in which many cells play a role, in particular mast cells, eosinophils, and T lymphocytes. In susceptible individuals this inflammation causes recurrent episodes of wheezing, breathlessness, chest tightness, and cough particularly at night and or in the early morning. These symptoms are usually associated with widespread but variable airflow limitation that is at least partly reversible either spontaneously or with treatment. The inflammation also causes an associated increase in airway responsiveness to a variety of stimuli."

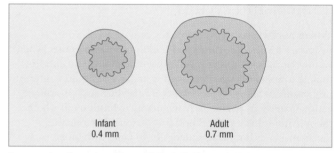

Infant
0.4 mm

Adult
0.7 mm

Comparative diameters of bronchioles in infant and adult

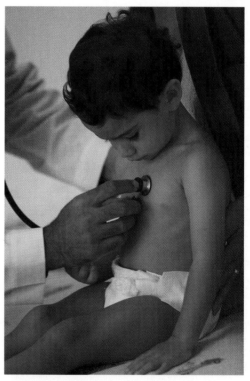

A definition of asthma

In the UK about 1.6 million children aged 2-15 have asthma symptoms that require treatment

of the immunology of asthma, hint at the possibility of factors either in utero or in early life that might modify an individual's atopic tendency.

The ISAAC study suggested that asthma prevalence was not directly related to air pollution. Regions such as China and Eastern Europe, with high levels of particulate matter and sulphur dioxide pollution, had low rates of asthma, whereas Western Europe and the US, with high levels of ozone, had an intermediate prevalence of asthma. Centres with the lowest levels of air pollution, such as New Zealand, had a high prevalence of asthma.

The International Study Asthma and Allergies in Childhood (ISAAC) attempted to identify further important environmental risk factors in the pathogenesis of asthma and related atopic disorders, being a population based study spanning 56 countries with 155 centres taking part. Nearly half a million children aged 13-14 completed a written questionnaire on symptoms of asthma, allergic conjunctivitis, and atopic eczema; over 300 000 completed a video questionnaire. The highest prevalence asthma symptoms was from the UK, New Zealand, and Australia, with a consistently high prevalence of other atopic disorders such as eczema and hay fever

---

Public health issues

In terms of burden of disease, childhood asthma presents a serious public health problem. More than half of all cases of asthma present before the age of 10, and over 30% of children experience a wheezing illness during the first few years of life. More absence from school is caused by asthma than any other chronic condition; 30% of asthmatic children miss more than three weeks of schooling each year. Asthma influences educational attainment even in children of above average intelligence, the extent of this adverse effect being related to severity of the disease.

Reasons for the increasing prevalence

It is unlikely that there is a single cause and effect association to account for the rise in prevalence of asthma and atopic disorders. Recent immunological studies, however, have indicated that the first three years of life (including life before birth) are probably the most critical in terms of environmental influences on the development of the asthma phenotype. For example, there are strong links between cigarette smoking in pregnancy and narrow airways in the offspring, and the risk of a child developing asthma is more closely associated with allergy in the mother than in the father.

Changes such as those in housing that allow proliferation of house dust mite, the effects of outdoor and indoor pollutants such as cigarette smoke, dietary changes, and low birth weight and prematurity may all account for some of the increased prevalence. To account for the increase in disease prevalence from 10% to 15% (such as has occurred in the UK over the past 30 years), however, the proportion of the population exposed to these hazards would need to have increased from 10% to nearly 70%, suggesting that other, as yet unidentified, risk factors may be operating.

The relevance of atopy

Atopy, defined as the predisposition to raise specific IgE to common allergens, is probably the single strongest risk factor for asthma, carrying up to a 20-fold increased risk of asthma in atopic individuals compared with non-atopic individuals. The

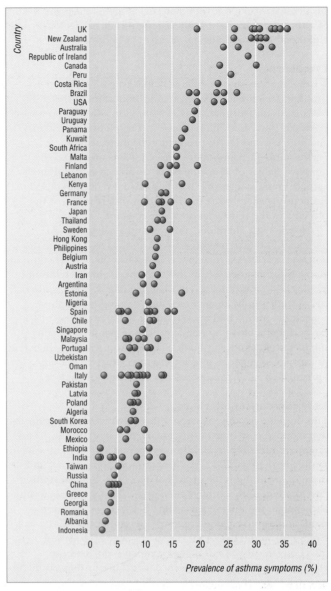

Prevalence of self reported asthma symptoms from written questionnaires (12 month period). Data from Office of Population, Censuses and Surveys. *Mortality Statistics 1990–92.* London: HMSO

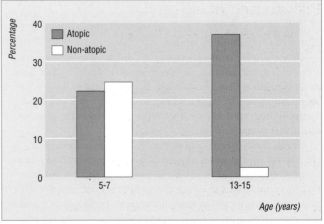

Atopy in children with bronchial hyperreactivity

strongest association is with maternal atopy—a maternal history of asthma or rhinitis, or both, is a significant risk factor for late childhood onset asthma and recurrent wheezing.

Lymphocytes

T lymphocytes—in particular T helper type 2 (Th2) lymphocytes—are also believed to be important in the pathogenesis of asthma. The fetal immune system is primarily polarised towards a Th2 response as a result of interleukin 4 and 10 (IL-4 and IL-10) production by the placenta. Furthermore, T lymphocytes isolated from cord blood of newborn babies of atopic mothers are able to respond to aeroallergens, suggesting that they may have been exposed to antigens ingested by the mother and transferred across the placenta in the third trimester of pregnancy.

During early childhood, environmental allergens—in particular intestinal microflora—are thought to influence the immune deviation of T helper cells towards the Th1 type in non-atopic children and towards the Th2 type in atopic children. In atopic children with recurrent wheezing illness, bronchoalveolar lavage studies indicate increased mast cell and eosinophil concentrations in children as young as 3. Up to the age of 10, the peripheral blood mononuclear cell response to specific stimulation in children who develop atopic disease is deficient in its capacity to generate interferon gamma, thereby causing upregulation of Th2 responses and an allergic phenotype.

Early exposure to infections

The "hygiene hypothesis" argues that the increase in asthma is due to a decrease in exposure to infection in early life. Frequent infections in childhood generate Th1 cytokines such as the interleukins IL-12, IL-18, and interferon gamma, and these in turn inhibit the growth of Th2 cells, thus preventing development of the asthma phenotype. The hypothesis would also explain the inverse association between socioeconomic status and asthma and allergy, with the assumption that children from higher social classes are exposed to fewer infections in early life. It may also explain why firstborn children have a higher prevalence of asthma, as they would be exposed to fewer infections from siblings.

Prospects for prevention

Allergen avoidance studies—such as the Isle of Wight study, in which infants born to mothers with a strong family history of atopy were randomised to receive prophylaxis with the mother eating a hypoallergenic diet and breast feeding or giving a soya milk preparation to their babies—showed a significant decrease in the prevalence of eczema and reactions to skin prick tests to aeroallergens and dietary factors, but no sustained benefit in relation to reduction in asthma.

Other similar studies focusing on dietary manipulation to prevent atopic eczema have shown equivocal results, but breast feeding is still advised in children from atopic families or in babies identified by high concentration of IgE in cord blood. Breastfeeding mothers are also advised to avoid allergens to which they are sensitive.

These results seem to indicate that the development of asthma is a combination of genetic susceptibility and exposure in early life to allergic stimuli and pollutants that augment a Th2 immune response. Once the asthma is established, cycles of acute and chronic inflammation triggered by allergens, viruses, pollutants, diet, and stress are responsible for exacerbations.

Recent studies indicate that the rise in childhood obesity may also be linked with the rise in childhood asthma. The

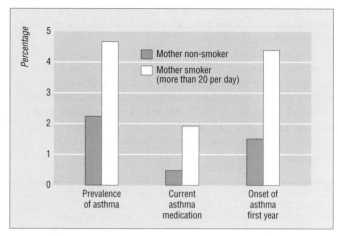

Maternal smoking and asthma in 4331 children aged 0-5, based on NHS interview survey

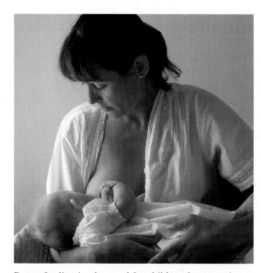

Exposure to relevant allergens in infancy or childhood may predispose a person to continued allergic responses later

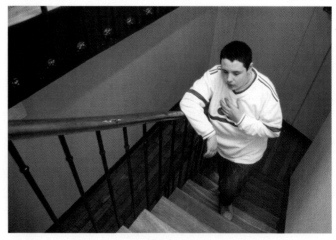

Breast feeding is advocated for children from atopic families. With permission from Ron Sutherland/Science Photo Library

Childhood obesity may be linked to an increase in childhood asthma. With permission from BSIP, Laurent/Science Photo Library

fattest children were more likely to have symptoms of asthma, suggesting that increased weight might lead to a risk of inflammation in the respiratory tract or might hinder respiratory flow.

Primary preventive measures to reduce risk might therefore include allergen avoidance, cessation of smoking, and attenuation of a Th2 response by vaccination. Once asthma is established, however, T cells and eosinophil responses may have enhanced capacity to generate the leukotrienes IL-3, IL-4, and IL-5, and it may be more difficult to reverse an established Th2 response. In this situation, secondary prevention measures to reduce exposure to trigger factors are appropriate.

Trigger factors in asthma

- Viral infections
- Dusts and pollutants including cigarette smoke
- Allergens—for example, house dust mite, pollens, moulds, spores, animal dander and feathers, certain foods, *Alternaria* in dry arid conditions
- Exercise
- Changes in weather patterns and cold air
- Psychological factors such as stress and emotion

Trigger factors in asthma

During the preschool years viral infections, exercise, and emotional upset are all common triggers of asthma. Young children contract six to eight viral upper respiratory tract infections each year so it is not surprising that these infections are more common precipitants of asthma in children than in adults. Asthmatic children tend to have more symptoms during the winter than the summer, probably because viral respiratory infections are more common in winter and because exercise induced asthma is more likely to develop outdoors in cold weather.

The domestic environment

If asthmatic children are sensitised to house dust mite parents can reduce exposure by removing carpets or vacuum cleaning regularly and dusting surfaces with damp cloths, as well as encasing mattresses and pillows in plastic sheets, washing covers, blankets, duvets, and furry toys regularly, and applying acaricides to soft furnishings. A recent Cochrane review, however, suggests that chemical and physical measures to reduce house dust mite cannot be recommended on the basis of the evidence available.

Smoking

Tobacco smoke has consistently been found to trigger exacerbation of asthma in children, and families should be encouraged to stop smoking or smoke in areas away from children outside the house. In addition, in families with a strong family history of asthma, and in children exposed to maternal smoking during pregnancy, there is a fourfold risk of developing wheezing illnesses in young children.

Air pollution

Epidemiological studies have suggested that certain types of outdoor air pollution (sulphur dioxide and high diesel particulates) may provoke emergency admissions for asthma or aggravate existing chronic asthma.

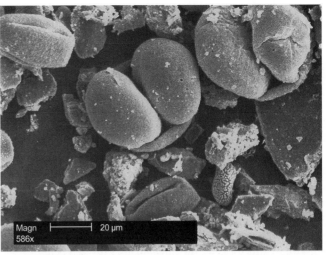

Electron micrograph of pollen grains. (Center for Disease Control)

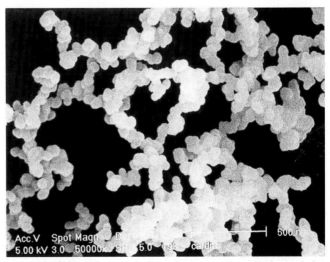

Vacuuming and other measures can make a house more bearable for children with asthma (Cristina Pedrazzini/Science Photo Library)

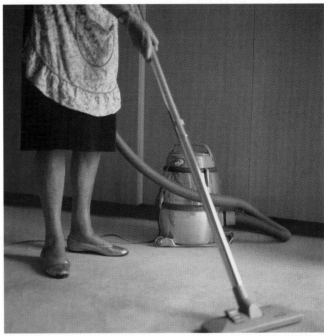

Electron micrograph of diesel particles. Photograph courtesy of Professor RJ Richards, Cardiff University. Published in Snashall D, Patel D (eds). *ABC of Occupational and Environmental Medicine*. 2nd ed. Oxford: Blackwell Publishing, 2003

Intervention

Tertiary prevention includes the provision of up to date guidelines to improve bronchodilation, reduce inflammation, and improve quality of life. In addition, airway remodelling may occur early in the course of disease and may then lead to irreversible loss of pulmonary function. The early administration of topical steroids may modify this development.

Airway inflammation

Fibreoptic bronchoscopy, biopsy, and bronchoalveolar lavage in the airways of asthmatic adults have shown that there is an inflammatory cellular infiltrate even when they are free of symptoms. This has led to the concept that asthma is a chronic inflammatory disorder. Eosinophils and mast cells are the important effector cells, the inflammatory process being modulated by T lymphocytes and macrophages and amplified by neural mechanisms.

Indirect evidence of an inflammatory process in the airways of young children has come from measurement of markers of inflammation in the blood and bronchoalveolar lavage, but few histological studies are available in children. The airways of children who have died from asthma, however, have shown an intense inflammatory response. We do not know how or when the inflammatory process starts, at what stage it becomes irreversible, or even whether the same type of inflammatory response occurs in all young wheezy children.

No component of the inflammatory process can be used as a diagnostic test for childhood asthma or as a reliable way to assess response to treatment. Diagnosis and the choice of treatment still depend on clinical judgment based on the nature, frequency, and severity of symptoms combined with physiological assessment of airway function.

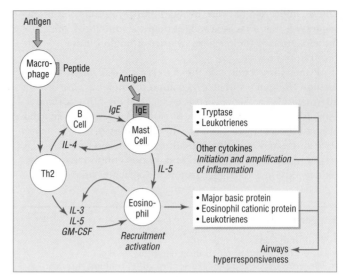

Mechanisms of mast cell and eosinophil dependent airway hyperresponsiveness. Adapted from Drazen JM, et al. *J Exp Med* 1996; 183:1-5

Further reading

- Aberg N, Hesselmar B, Aberg B, Eriksson B. Increase of asthma, allergic rhinitis and eczema in Swedish schoolchildren between 179 and 1991. *Clin Exp Allergy* 1995;25:815-19.
- Akinbami LJ, Schoendorf KC. Trends in childhood asthma: prevalence, health care utilization, and mortality. *Pediatrics* 2002;110:315-22.
- Custovic A, Simpson A, Chapman MD, Woodcock A. Allergen avoidance in the treatment of asthma and atopic disorders. *Thorax* 1998;53:63-72.
- Dezateux C, Stocks J, Dundas I, Fletcher ME. Impaired airway function and wheezing in infancy: the influence of maternal smoking and a genetic predisposition to asthma. *Am J Respir Crit Care Med* 1999;159:403-10.
- Drazen JM, Arm JP, Austen KF. Sorting out the cytokines of asthma. *J Exp Med* 1996;183:1-5.
- Gdalevich M, Mimouni D, Mimouni M. Breast-feeding and the risk of bronchial asthma in childhood: a systematic review with meta-analysis of prospective studies. *J Pediatr* 2001;139:261-6.
- Godden DJ, Ross S, Abdalla M, McMurray D, Douglas A, Oldman D, *et al.* Outcome of wheeze in childhood. *Am J Respir Crit Care Med* 1994;149:106-12.
- Gotzsche PC, Johansen HK, Schmidt LM, Burr ML. House dust mite control measures for asthma. *Cochrane Database Syst Rev* 2005;(2):CD001187.
- Hide DW, Matthews S, Tariq S, Arshad SH. Allergen avoidance in infancy and allergy at 4 years of age. *Allergy* 1996;51:89–93.
- Holt PG, Clough JB, Holt BJ, Baron-Hay MJ, Rose AH, Robinson BW, et al. Genetic "risk" for atopy is associated with delayed postnatal maturation of T cell competence. *Clin Exp Allergy* 1992;22:1093-9.
- International Consensus Report on the Diagnosis and Management of Asthma. *Clin Exper Allergy* 1992;22(suppl 1).
- ISAAC Steering Committee. Worldwide variation in prevalence of symptoms of asthma, allergic conjunctivitis, and atopic eczema: ISAAC. *Lancet* 1998:351:1225-31.
- Figueroa-Muñoz JI, Chinn S, Rona RJ. Association between obesity and asthma in 4–11 year old children in the UK. *Thorax* 2001;56:133-7.
- Russell G, Helms PJ. Trends in occurrence of asthma among children and young adults. *BMJ* 1997;315:1014-5.

12 Patterns of illness and diagnosis

Wheezing in infancy

Young children up to the age of 3 are particularly prone to wheezing illnesses. Researchers have differentiated early transient wheezers from persistent wheezers by analysis of risk factors and lung function tests. The transient wheezers had smaller airways and their mothers smoked, whereas the persistent wheezers had a more classic atopic history with a positive family history of maternal asthma, raised serum IgE, and positive results to skin prick tests.

Respiratory tract infections

Many babies have repeated episodes of wheezing associated with viral respiratory tract infections. The mechanism by which this happens is still not fully understood, but genetic constitution and environmental influences in early life may predispose to wheeze by causing changes in airway calibre or in lung function. For example, wheezy lower respiratory illnesses are more common among boys, among infants of parents who smoke, and among babies born prematurely who have needed prolonged positive pressure ventilation. Thus pre-existing factors other than asthma that cause narrowing of the airways account for more than half of the wheezing developed by infants.

Bronchiolitis

About 1% of infants are admitted to hospital with acute viral bronchiolitis. Recurrent cough and wheezing commonly follow but in most cases stop before school age. About 40% of babies with atopic eczema also develop recurrent wheezing, and there is a strong association between a family history of atopic disease and wheezing in early childhood. According to data from Martinez and colleagues (see box) 14% of children had persistent wheezing from infancy to the age of 6 (persistent wheezers), and this group also had the highest proportion of viral respiratory disease in the first year of life, suggesting that some viral infections may facilitate the development of asthma, whereas others (as discussed in chapter 11) may help to modify the immune response in such a way as to protect against asthma.

Progression of asthma from childhood to adolescence

The outcome of early onset wheeze is still controversial. Children seen in referral centres have poorer outcomes than those followed up in longitudinal studies of general populations, probably because those with more severe asthma are referred to hospital.

Predictability

The data from Martinez and colleagues would suggest that early onset asthma is associated with poor outcome in terms of lung function and persistent bronchial hyperresponsiveness. Another study in infants aged 1 month showed that those who were more responsive to histamine challenge were more likely to have asthma diagnosed at the age of 6, and other studies have shown a clear relation between degree of airway

A prospective study by Martinez and colleagues in 1995 looked at over 1200 children born in Tucson, Arizona. By the age of 6, 826 children (51%) had never wheezed. Three patterns were identified in the others: 20% of children who had wheezed early on with respiratory tract infections had no wheezing by the age of 6 (early transient group), 15% had no wheezing at the age of 3 but had wheezing at the age of 6 (late onset group), and 14% had wheezing before the age of 3 and at the age of 6 (persistent wheezers)

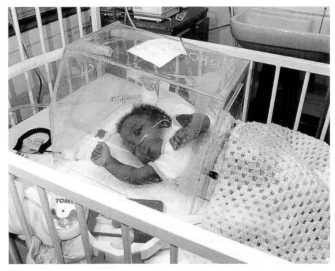

About 1% of infants will be admitted to hospital with acute viral bronchiolitis

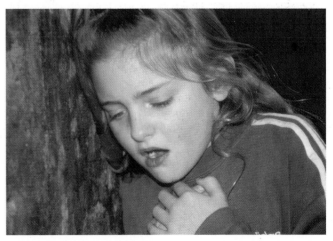

With permission from Mark Clarke/Science Photo Library

hyperresponsiveness to histamine challenge and persistence of asthma.

In a review of patients aged 29-32 who had previously been studied at the age of 7 by questionnaire and spirometry, however, Jenkins and colleagues found that of those who had reported asthma at age 7, only 26% still had symptoms as adults. Other childhood risk factors that predicted asthma in adult life included being female, a family history of asthma, and more severe asthma (especially if it developed after the age of 2 and was associated with reduced expiratory flow rate).

A population study in New Zealand reported that as children grow older bronchial hyperreactivity decreases. Judged by the response to inhaled histamine, the number of children with hyperresponsive airways halved between the ages of 6 and 12. In contrast, the total number of children with atopy doubled. Of those aged 5-7 who had evidence of bronchial reactivity, about half were atopic; of the children aged 13 with bronchial hyperresponsiveness over 90% were atopic.

Results of studies

These results support the clinical observations that non-specific factors—notably viral infections and exercise—are important triggers of asthma during preschool years, and allergic triggers assume greater importance as children grow older. Other similar longitudinal studies suggest that children with mild disease usually outgrow their asthma as a result of the increase in airway size with growth and the apparent spontaneous decline in airway responsiveness with age. However, females and those with more severe disease, greater airway hyperresponsiveness, and an atopic history tend to have more persistent disease.

Teenagers with asthma

Asthmatic teenagers are coping with a period of intense emotional and psychological change, and this can have a considerable impact on quality of life. They also have concerns about body image, peer acceptance, physical capabilities in terms of exercise and activity, and the physiological delay of puberty caused by their asthma, all of which can complicate their asthma treatment goals.

In addition, because of a need to emphasise their own identity, they may become isolated and may experience anxiety and depression, especially if they are excluded from participation in the decision making process regarding their condition. They may also participate in risky behaviour such as cigarette smoking and non-compliance with treatment, which may account for their increased morbidity and mortality.

In 2000, annual hospital admission rates for asthma were 48 per 10 000 children aged <5 and 16 per 10 000 children aged 5-14. Between 1990 and 2000, hospital admission rates had decreased by 52% among children <5 and by 45% among children aged 5-14. The weekly incidence of acute asthma attacks diagnosed by a general practitioner increased markedly during the 1970s and 1980s, peaked in the early 1990s, and by 2000 declined quite substantially for the age groups <5 and 5-14. These are encouraging statistics and suggest that perhaps greater awareness of the problem, and better management guidelines have helped reduce the burden of disease for the population of UK teenagers.

Sympathetic consultation

Paediatricians need to recognise the needs of these vulnerable teenagers by spending more time listening to their requests, helping them to make choices about treatment, and negotiating a plan of action that allows for compromise on

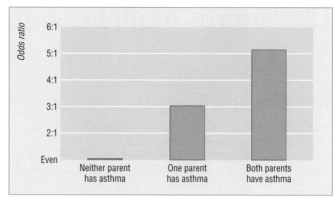

Odds ratios for asthma in children (from Weitzman M et al, *Pediatrics* 1990;85:505-11)

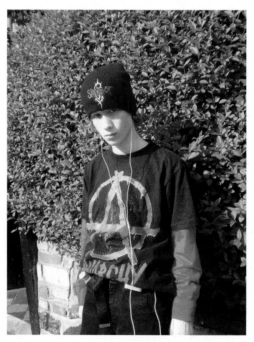

Asthma is often diagnosed in younger teenagers

The goals of treatment for teenagers with asthma are psychological wellbeing, full physical activity, and minimal effects on the underlying developmental progression from childhood to adulthood

both sides. Holding separate clinics for young people and being prepared to discuss wider issues other than asthma may go some way to improve understanding and compliance.

Diagnosis of asthma

The diagnosis of asthma is made after taking an appropriate clinical history and examination, testing for reversibility of bronchoconstriction and assessing a response to therapy. Demonstration of airway reversibility or a short term trial with antiasthma therapy may be useful diagnostic markers, especially in those children with episodic symptoms (see chapter 3 on peak flow variation, p.9).

Presentation

In school age children there is little difficulty in recognising asthma, especially when one asks specifically about cough, wheeze, shortness of breath, and exercise induced symptoms. Preschool children sometimes present with cough alone. The other characteristics that suggest asthma are episodic cough or wheeze and symptoms that are worse at night, after exercise or exposure to allergens, and with viral respiratory tract infections. Asthmatic babies sometimes have attacks of breathlessness without obvious wheezing.

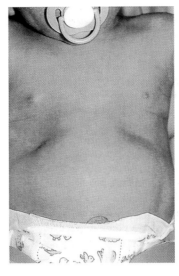

Chest deformity like this is an indication to treat with inhaled steroids

Hypersecretory asthma

Some asthmatic children produce large amounts of bronchial secretions. This is called hypersecretory asthma. Increased production of mucus is associated with a productive cough, airway plugging, and areas of collapse on the chest radiograph. These children may be misdiagnosed as having recurrent lower respiratory tract infection.

Most wheezing in infancy is due to accumulation of secretions in the airway in response to bronchial inflammation. Certain features, however, suggest that the cough or wheezing may be caused by factors other than asthma. These include onset soon after birth, chronic diarrhoea or failure to thrive, recurrent infections, a persistent wet cough, stridor, choking or difficulty with swallowing, mediastinal or focal abnormalities on the chest radiograph, and the presence of cardiovascular abnormalities.

Other causes of noisy breathing in children

- Bronchiolitis
- Inhalation—such as foreign body, milk
- Gastro-oesophageal reflux
- Cystic fibrosis
- Ciliary dyskinesia
- Laryngeal problem
- Tuberculosis
- Bronchomalacia
- Tracheal/bronchial stenosis
- Vascular rings
- Mediastinal masses

Lung function and other tests

When possible the diagnosis should be confirmed by lung function testing. This can be done at any age, but in infants and very young children the facilities are available only in specialised centres. From the age of 4 some children can use a peak flow meter, and the peak flow reading can be compared with a range of values related to the child's height. A normal peak flow reading at one examination does not exclude asthma and several recordings made at home may be more valuable. If the result of spirometry is normal, then reversibility testing is of little use. Occasionally an exercise test or therapeutic trial is necessary to confirm the diagnosis. Measurement of total IgE concentration will ascertain only whether the child is atopic. A chest radiograph is more useful to look for other causes of wheezing than to diagnose asthma.

Labelling

Making a diagnosis of asthma carries with it a certain stigma, for no parent likes to be told their child may have a chronic illness with the possibility of recurrent exacerbations. With appropriate explanation and reassurance, however, parental anxiety is more likely to be reduced and compliance with therapy increased.

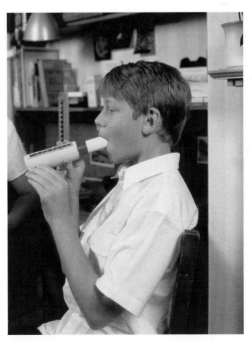

A peak flow meter can be used by some children (over 4 years) to test lung function. With permission of Mark Clark/Science Photo Library

Assessment of severity

Ideally the management of asthma should include serial measurement of markers of disease activity, but as yet there are none that can be applied to the clinical care of asthmatic children. Evaluation of severity and response to treatment has therefore to be made by clinical assessment complemented when possible by measurements of peak flow and lung function. A sound approach is to classify the asthma as mild, moderate, or severe; to base the initial treatment regimen on this assessment; and then decide at regular reviews whether there is scope to modify medication.

Mild asthma—For asthma to be categorised as mild, symptomatic episodes should occur less often than once a month. Symptoms do not interfere with daytime activity or sleep. There is a good response to bronchodilator treatment, and lung function returns to normal between attacks.

Moderate asthma—Children with moderate asthma have some symptoms several days a week and have attacks of asthma more than once a month but less than once a week. There is no chest deformity and growth is unaffected. Attacks may be triggered by viral infection, allergens, exercise, cigarette smoke, climatic changes, and emotional upset.

Severe asthma—The third category, severe asthma, is the least common. Children have troublesome symptoms on most days, wake frequently with asthma at night, miss school, and are unable to participate fully in school or outdoor activities. Their growth may be retarded, and they may have chest deformities.

Some children do not fit any of these categories. Seasonal asthma caused by allergy to grass pollen generally affects older children. A few children have sudden very severe attacks of asthma, which result in admission to hospital and may be life threatening, separated by long periods without symptoms during which their lung function returns to normal. This latter group are difficult to treat.

Further reading
- Gerritsen J, Koeter GH, Postma DS, Schouten JP, van Aalderen WM, Knol K. Airway responsiveness in childhood as a predictor of the outcome of asthma in adulthood. *Am Rev Respir Dis* 1991;143:1468-9.
- Jenkins MA, Hopper JL, Bowes G, Carlin JB, Flander LB, Giles GG. Factors in childhood as predictors of asthma in adult life. *BMJ* 1994;309:90-3.
- Martinez, FD, Wright AL, Taussig LM, Holberg CJ, Halonen M, Margan WJ. Asthma and wheezing in the first six years of life. The Group Health Medical Associates. *N Engl J Med* 1995;332:133-8.
- *Health survey for England*. London: Department of Health, 1996, 1997.
- Roorda RJ. Prognostic factors for the outcome of childhood asthma in adolescence. *Thorax* 1996;51(suppl 1):S7-12.

13 Treatment

There are several non-pharmacological therapies for the management of paediatric asthma, some of which have been discussed in earlier chapters. These include measures to avoid allergens and reduction of exposure to cigarette smoke. Cochrane reviews of other therapies, including complementary therapies, have shown some beneficial effect in the general wellbeing of the patient but no direct benefit in terms of asthma symptoms.

Pharmacological management

The aims of treatment can be achieved by prompt diagnosis, identification of trigger factors, evaluation of severity, establishment of a partnership of management with the asthmatic child and the family, and regular review.

Partnership in management

Self management plans allow a partnership to be established between the doctor, the child, and his or her family. The aim of the plan is to allow families to become more confident about the day-to-day management of asthma, to cope with exacerbations, and to prevent hospital admission with early intervention and thereby ultimately reduce health costs.

In young children, plans are based on the child's symptoms and less so on objective assessments such as peak flow measurements. In older children, peak flow assessments are useful, especially for those who are poor perceivers of symptoms.

Respiratory nurses working in asthma clinics, schools, and general practice have a pivotal role in establishing this partnership. They also keep in regular personal contact and reassure and encourage children and their families. In addition, there is a wealth of information available from organisations such as Asthma UK.

Changing the environment

As mentioned earlier, the avoidance of cigarette smoking is important especially during pregnancy. Families with asthmatic children should be discouraged from acquiring pets. With a pet already present, the pet allergy has to be established with a good history of exacerbation after contact, as well as skin prick tests or specific IgE levels, before removal is advised. It may take several months before the animal dander completely disappears. There is some evidence, however, that maintaining exposure to cat allergen in the domestic environment might induce tolerance of the immune system.

House dust mite

House dust mite sensitivity is the most common allergy in asthmatic children. At high altitudes where concentrations of house dust mite and other inhaled antigens are low, symptoms, bronchial reactivity and the need for medication are considerably reduced. Only considerable environmental changes to reduce house dust mite, however, have been shown to be effective in improving asthma.

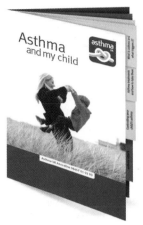 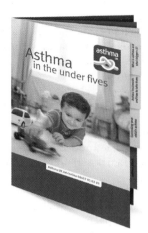

Asthma UK produce useful leaflets for parents of newly diagnosed children and those who are living with asthma (available from www.asthma.org.uk)

The aims of treatment should be:

- To control symptoms and allow children to lead a full and active life at home and at school
- To restore normal lung function and reduce variations in peak flow
- To minimise the requirement for bronchodilator therapy and prevent exacerbations
- To enable normal growth and development and avoid adverse effects of medication

---

The outcomes of successful self management are:

- Absence of or minimal cough, shortness of breath, and wheeze, including nocturnal symptoms
- Minimal or infrequent exacerbations
- Minimal need for bronchodilator therapy
- No limitation of activity, especially exercise and games
- Restoration of normal lung function and reduce variations in peak flow
- Minimal or no adverse effects of the medications

Partnership comprises:

- An understanding of asthma and goals of treatment
- Monitoring of symptoms
- Use of a peak flow meter when appropriate
- An agreed plan of action of what to do when the child's asthma improves, gets worse, or there is an acute attack
- Clear written instructions

Asthma UK is a charity dedicated to improving the health and wellbeing of people in the UK whose lives are affected by asthma
Website: www.asthma.org.uk
Advice line: 08457 01 02 03

Further reading

- Platts-Mills T, Vaughan J, Squillace S, Woodfolk J, Sporik R. Sensitisation, asthma, and a modified TH2 response in children exposed to cat allergen: a population-based cross-sectional study. *Lancet* 2001;357:752-6.

14 Drug treatment

The British Guideline on the Management of Asthma (2003) proposes a stepwise and algorithmic approach to drug management in paediatric asthma.

Bronchodilators

Children with mild episodic asthma need only intermittent treatment with short acting bronchodilator drugs, which should be given whenever possible by inhalation (step 1 of the guidelines). Those with more severe asthma who are taking a prophylactic agent should always have a short acting bronchodilator readily available. The selective β_2 adrenergic agonists (for example, salbutamol and terbutaline) are the best and safest bronchodilators. Asthma in childhood is often triggered by viral respiratory tract infections and exercise. It may be necessary to take a bronchodilator as required during and for a week or two after a cold. A single dose of an inhaled β_2 adrenergic bronchodilator taken 15-20 minutes before a games period at school can also help to prevent exercise induced wheezing.

Children who often use their bronchodilator more than three times a week should be reviewed with a view to additional preventive therapy.

Prophylactic agents

The biggest advance in the treatment of asthma came with the development of topically active inhaled corticosteroids. Non-steroidal prophylactic agents include long acting β_2 agonists, leukotriene antagonists, and theophyllines.

Lung function between attacks can be assessed by spirometric measurements of FEV_1 and forced vital capacity (FVC). More subtle abnormalities can be detected by forced expiratory flow volume curves or by measurement of lung volumes in a respiratory function laboratory.

A single measurement of peak expiratory flow rate (PEFR) may be misleading, but recordings made at home in the morning and afternoon or evening over a week or two may show variations that indicate airway instability and the need for prophylactic medication. Once started, regular treatment with a prophylactic agent is likely to be needed for years rather than months and should be withdrawn only when there has been little need for bronchodilator treatment for at least three months. Close supervision is necessary during withdrawal of a prophylactic drug.

Inhaled steroids

Corticosteroids are the most potent anti-inflammatory agents available for treating asthma, and they have the greatest diversity of action.

Dose
The starting dose depends on clinical assessment of severity, and in older children with frequent symptoms it may be appropriate to start with a moderate dose of inhaled corticosteroid together with a long acting β_2 adrenergic agonist

---

Important points to remember when following the guidelines

- There is a stepwise approach to asthma management for children aged 5-12 and children aged <5
- Children should start at the step most appropriate to the severity of presentation of asthma and then move up or down the steps until a minimal effective dose of inhaled steroid is achieved to control symptoms
- Before stepping up at any stage of treatment, ensure compliance is good, that an appropriate inhaler device is given, and that technique is good. Exclude other possible diagnoses such as gastro-oesophageal reflux, bronchiolitis, inhalation of foreign body, and cystic fibrosis
- A rescue course of prednisolone 1-2 mg/kg/day at any step is allowed for three to five days for acute exacerbations without the requirement for dose tapering; a short acting bronchodilator can also be used more often during and after such exacerbations
- Children with chronic asthma should be reviewed every three to six months and, if they are stable, advised to reduce the dose of inhaled steroid by 25-50% until a minimum effective dose is achieved

---

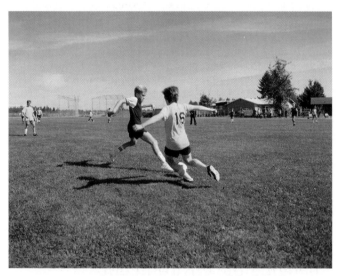

A single dose of an inhaled β_2 adrenergic bronchodilator can help to prevent exercise-induced wheezing (photos.com)

When to consider regular prophylactic medication

- Frequent symptoms and the need to take a bronchodilator several days a week
- Frequent nocturnal cough and wheezing even without troublesome asthma during the day
- At least one asthma attack a month
- Lung function fails to return to normal between attacks

Indications for prescribing inhaled steroids to children

- As first line prophylactic therapy (step 2)
- Moderate asthma, recurrent acute attacks, daily wheeze and shortness of breath
- When asthma is more severe (step 3 or step 4), particularly in those children with chest deformity

and then reduce the dose of steroid in a stepwise fashion to the minimum effective dose required to prevent symptoms (stepping down).

Methods of delivery

Inhaled steroids given by pressurised aerosol (pMDI) or by dry powder inhaler are effective in older children. Inhaled steroids have also been used increasingly to treat asthma in preschool children. Many children with recurrent viral induced wheeze, however, do not go on to develop atopic asthma and probably would not benefit from long term inhaled corticosteroid prophylaxis.

When an inhaled steroid is given to a preschool child with frequent or severe asthma through a spacer with a one way valve and a face mask, it is as effective as in older children; and this seems to be the best delivery system.

Inhaled steroid (budesonide or beclometasone) is usually started at a dose of 200-400 μg/day in children and fluticasone is given at half this dose (that is, 100-200 μg/day).

Trials of steroids given by nebuliser to young children in conventional doses (200-400 μg/day) have given disappointing results. This is probably because the amount of drug delivered in a suspension from a nebuliser to a freely breathing infant or young child is small. Over three quarters of the drug remains in the nebuliser and fewer than 20% of the nebulised droplets containing the drug are <5 μm diameter. To overcome this problem it is necessary to use large starting doses. Doses of nebulised budesonide up to 1000 μg/day have shown a therapeutic effect in infants with severe asthma.

Adverse effects

There is a reluctance to give inhaled and oral steroids to young children because of possible side effects. Local side effects such as oral thrush and dysphonia are rare in children, probably because powder inhalers and spacer devices are used.

It is difficult to separate the adverse effects of asthma from the adverse effects of inhaled corticosteroids on children's growth. Likewise, if children whose asthma is well controlled on low dose steroids are placed on high dose steroids, growth may be stunted, whereas children with severe asthma may not experience any adverse effects but instead may enjoy a good period of growth as a result of better control.

Evidence on the effects of inhaled corticosteroids on growth shows that both beclometasone and budesonide at doses used at step 3 or above of the BTS guidelines affect childhood growth as assessed by knemometry (leg length below the knee) and conventional stadiometry. Studies have not, however, shown any adverse effect on final height.

The exact mechanism of the adverse effect of inhaled steroids on growth is unknown but is believed to be the result of decreased bone turnover rather than changes in growth hormone or IGF1 levels. The effects of inhaled corticosteroids on bone mineral density are more worrying because they are cumulative. Long term inhaled corticosteroids may be inducing a state of bone demineralisation that could lead to osteoporosis in the long term, particularly in women.

Some studies have identified symptomatic adrenal insufficiency in children on high dosages of inhaled corticosteroids. A recent study by Masoli and colleagues suggests that therapeutic gain at high doses of inhaled corticosteroids >800 μg/day is likely to be small—the so called "ceiling effect"—and therefore the clinician has to exclude other causes of treatment failure, such as poor adherence to treatment and alternative diagnoses, before using higher doses of inhaled corticosteroids as recommended at step 4.

A few children on high doses of inhaled steroid have clinical

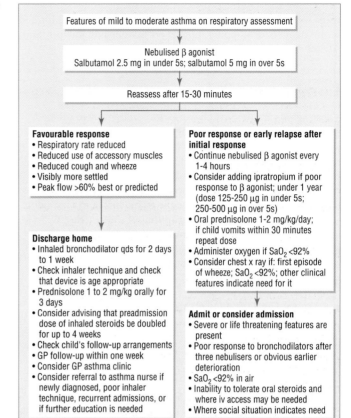

Features of mild to moderate asthma on respiratory assessment

↓

Nebulised β agonist
Salbutamol 2.5 mg in under 5s; salbutamol 5 mg in over 5s

↓

Reassess after 15-30 minutes

Favourable response
- Respiratory rate reduced
- Reduced use of accessory muscles
- Reduced cough and wheeze
- Visibly more settled
- Peak flow >60% best or predicted

Discharge home
- Inhaled bronchodilator qds for 2 days to 1 week
- Check inhaler technique and check that device is age appropriate
- Prednisolone 1 to 2 mg/kg orally for 3 days
- Consider advising that preadmission dose of inhaled steroids be doubled for up to 4 weeks
- Check child's follow-up arrangements
- GP follow-up within one week
- Consider GP asthma clinic
- Consider referral to asthma nurse if newly diagnosed, poor inhaler technique, recurrent admissions, or if further education is needed

Poor response or early relapse after initial response
- Continue nebulised β agonist every 1-4 hours
- Consider adding ipratropium if poor response to β agonist; under 1 year (dose 125-250 μg in under 5s; 250-500 μg in over 5s)
- Oral prednisolone 1-2 mg/kg/day; if child vomits within 30 minutes repeat dose
- Administer oxygen if SaO₂ <92%
- Consider chest x ray if: first episode of wheeze; SaO₂ <92%; other clinical features indicate need for it

Admit or consider admission
- Severe or life threatening features are present
- Poor response to bronchodilators after three nebulisers or obvious earlier deterioration
- SaO₂ <92% in air
- Inability to tolerate oral steroids and where iv access may be needed
- Where social situation indicates need

Management of mild to moderate exacerbations of asthma in children. Adapted from guidelines from the British Thoracic Society and Scottish Intercollegiate Guidelines Network

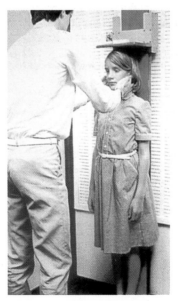

Stadiometry can be used to measure growth in children

adrenal insufficiency and present with hypoglycaemic episodes, coma, or convulsions. Patients and parents have to be reminded of the dangers of stopping inhaled corticosteroids abruptly and advised to seek medical advice when such events occur.

Long acting β_2 agonists

These agents are the first choice as add-on therapy to inhaled steroids in adults and children aged >4. They are available for paediatric usage at step 3 of the guidelines. In the UK, salmeterol is currently licensed for use in children from the age of 4 and formoterol in children age >6. They increase airway calibre for at least 12 hours, prevent exercise-induced symptoms for up to nine hours, and reduce the frequency of exacerbations.

Their safety profile is similar to that of short acting β_2 agonists. Although symptoms improve when these agents are given alone, their use is more appropriate in conjunction with regular anti-inflammatory therapy.

Leukotriene receptor antagonists

Leukotrienes are a recognised mediator of asthma as they cause bronchoconstriction, mucous secretion, and increased vascular permeability, promoting eosinophil migration into airways mucosa. Recent studies in children aged 6-14 treated with leukotriene receptor antagonists have shown an improvement in exercise induced bronchospasm and an improvement in FEV_1. Currently in the UK, montelukast (available in granules or as a pink, chewable, cherry flavoured tablet) is licensed for children aged >2 years and zafirlukast in those aged >12. These drugs are currently used at step 2 (children aged <5) or step 3 (children aged 5-12) in the management of paediatric asthma.

Sodium cromoglicate

Sodium cromoglicate is completely safe with virtually no side effects, even when it is taken regularly for years. Its taste and the requirement for it to be taken three or four times a day, however, makes non-compliance a common reason for failure of treatment. Furthermore, there is little evidence base for its use in the modern management of asthma.

Theophyllines

Theophylline can improve lung function and act as an effective bronchodilator with some anti-inflammatory action. Its safety margin is low compared with other bronchodilators and it is necessary to monitor treatment by serum concentration. It is important to bear in mind that barbiturates, carbamazepine, phenytoin, and rifamicin may reduce blood concentrations of xanthine derivatives and conversely cimetidine, erythromycin, and ciprofloxacin may increase these concentrations. Slow release granule preparations may suit some children.

Oral agents

When a drug has to be taken regularly there are potential advantages if it can be taken by mouth and only once or twice a day. Slow release theophylline in doses titrated to give blood concentrations of 10-20 mg/l will control asthma in children with frequent symptoms, but it is relatively ineffective in preventing the wheezing that accompanies viral upper respiratory tract infections. The variable clearance rate of

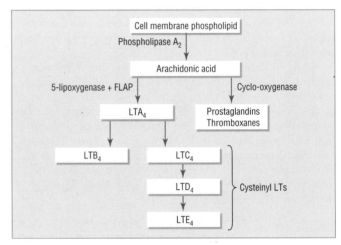

The leukotriene synthesis pathway. FLAP, 5-lipoxygenase activating protein

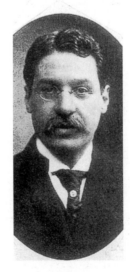

In 1900 Soloman Solis-Cohen reported the beneficial effects of oral dried bovine adrenal extract in 12 patients with asthma. This was probably the first recorded use of steroids in the treatment of asthma

theophylline in children means that it is difficult to predict the dose of the drug that will give therapeutic blood concentrations in an individual child.

Side effects of theophylline (notably, gastrointestinal upsets and behaviour disturbances) are common, particularly in preschool children. Because of problems with giving the drug and its side effects, use has been restricted to children whose asthma is uncontrolled despite treatment with inhaled steroids and where there has been no response to long acting β_2 agonists (step 3 add-on therapy).

Inhaler devices

Whenever possible asthma treatment should be given to children by inhalation, and the most common reasons for failure of inhaled treatment are inappropriate selection or incorrect use of the inhaler. Children become fully aware of their own breathing and recognise the difference between inspiration and expiration by about the age of 3; until then they need inhalation devices that require only tidal breathing. Inspiratory flow rates are slower and the airways narrower in children, and both these factors influence the dose inhaled and the site of deposition of the drug. The choice of inhaler will depend on the child's age and preference for a particular device.

Aerosols and powders

Hydrofluoroalkane (HFA) propellants are replacing chlorofluorocarbon (CFC) propellants in pressurised metered dose inhalers (pMDIs). Patients may notice a slight taste difference as a result and should be warned about this.

Most children under the age of 10 are unable to achieve the coordination needed to use an unmodified pMDI. Less than half of children obtain benefit from these devices because of poor inhalation technique. Breath actuated aerosol inhalers (Autohaler) are easier to use, but a child tends to close the glottis when the breath actuated valve opens and fewer children under the age of 7 are able to use these inhalers.

The age at which breath actuated dry powder inhalers such as the Accuhaler and Turbohaler can be used depends on the optimal inspiratory flow rate—for example, the Turbohaler needs an inspiration of about 30 l/minute. The latter can therefore be used in children over the age of 4-5 with proper training. In addition, twice as much drug can be deposited in the lungs with a Turbohaler than with the same drug given via a pMDI (without a spacer).

Spacers and nebulisers

A spacer device reduces the velocity of the particles before they reach the mouth and allows more of the propellant to evaporate so that the inhaled particles become smaller and penetrate further into the lungs. Recent developments include that of a metal spacer device, which has no electrostatic charge, no dead space, and may allow better lung deposition. After activation of the drug canister, the aerosol can be inhaled by taking a few breaths sufficient to open and close the valve attached to the mouthpiece. Children can use spacers in this way from the age of 2. Children under 2 can be given inhalers with a spacer and mask with the spacer held at 45° to keep the valve open. The infant can then inhale the medication during normal tidal respiration. During acute attacks, infants and young children may not tolerate a facemask, in which case only nebulised treatment is appropriate. Some parents report that their children cannot tolerate a facemask at all, and so a paper drinks carton can be used in place of a spacer.

Inhaler devices for children

	Age (years)		
	1-2	3-5	≥5
pMDI+spacer	1st choice	2nd choice	—
pMDI+spacer	2nd choice	1st choice	2nd choice
Breath actuated aerosol inhalers	Inappropriate	Useful	Equal 1st choice
Breath actuated dry powder inhaler	Inappropriate	Occasionally useful	Equal 1st choice

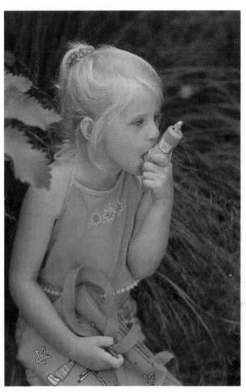

A 6 year old girl using a breath actuated aerosol inhaler (3M United Kingdom plc)

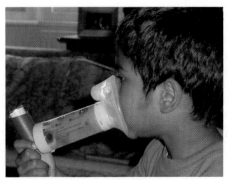

A 5 year old boy using a pMDI and spacer

The spacer should be cleaned when it becomes cloudy and at least once a month. The spacer should be washed in soapy water and left to air dry. Where possible they should be replaced every 6 to 12 months.

Nebulisers

Metered dose inhaler therapy with a spacer is at least as good as a nebuliser for treating mild and moderate exacerbations of asthma. In wheezy infants short acting β_2 adrenergic bronchodilators inhaled through a nebuliser may sometimes be associated with worsening of intrathoracic airway function: the poor response may be related to the small dose of drug reaching the airways. In young children the anticholinergic agent ipratropium bromide may be beneficial, given either through a nebuliser or a spacer device with a facemask.

Nebulisers are expensive, time consuming, and inconvenient. They are often used incorrectly at home. A compressor and jet nebuliser suitable for giving asthma medication should have a driving gas flow rate of 8-10 l/minute and a volume fill of 4 ml; this is particularly important when suspensions such as inhaled steroid are given. The equivalent dose for older children is not necessarily appropriate for a younger age group because inhalation technique, volume of tidal breathing, and the anatomy of the upper airway are different. Despite these reservations, however, there is an important place for the judicious use of nebulisers in the treatment of young asthmatic children at home. A double blind placebo controlled study of 36 children with poorly controlled asthma, showed a significant improvement in their asthma and reduction in intake of oral corticosteroids.

Choice of device

The patient's preference is of major importance in the choice of device. Many patients are unable to use pMDIs correctly, and even with good technique only 10-15% of the dose is delivered to the lungs.

Spacer devices will reduce problems with coordination and improve lung deposition. Children on regular prophylactic inhaled steroids are advised to use a spacer at all times. Even when a spacer device is used, correct positioning of the device, inhalation of the drug within 10-20 seconds, single dose actuations, and regular rinsing and drip drying of the spacer devices are important take home instructions.

Dry powder inhalers may also vary in their lung deposition, and up to 30% of a drug may reach the lungs with a good technique. The main determining factor for their use is variations in the inspiratory flow rate.

The future

Our understanding of the pathogenesis of childhood asthma continues to improve. However, we still need to identify more precisely those factors that can prevent the onset of disease and modify disease progression. Genetic markers should enable us to identify those children at risk, as well as allow more specific pharmacological therapies in individual cases.

Immunomodulation and modification of fetal and early life environmental factors are currently being evaluated, but in the meantime we need to improve both our and our patients' understanding of the disease, improve adherence to therapy, and continue to follow guidelines of management to minimise the potential side effects of therapy.

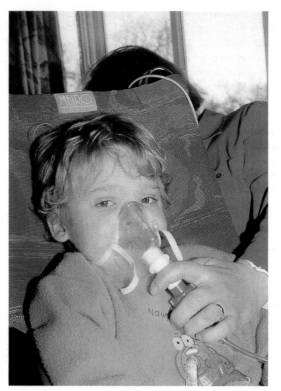

Nebulisers need to be used correctly in a domestic environment

When to refer to a specialist

- Uncertainty about the diagnosis
- Poor symptom control despite adequate therapy within guidelines
- Patient on high dosages of inhaled steroid (>800 μg/day)
- Parental concern/request for a second opinion
- Evidence of side effects

Further reading

- Agertoft L, Pedersen S. Effect of long-term treatment with inhaled budesonide on adult height on adult height in children with asthma. *N Engl J Med* 2000;343:1064-9.
- Ilangovan P, Pedersen S, Godfrey S, Nikander K, Noviski N, Warner JO. Treatment of severe steroid dependent pre-school asthma with nebulised budesonide suspension. *Arch Dis Child* 1993;68:356-9.
- Kemp JP, Dockhorn RJ, Shapiro GC, Nguyen HH, Reiss TF, Seidenberg BC, et al. Montelukast once daily inhibits exercise-induced bronchoconstriction in 6- to 14-year-old children with asthma. *J Pediatr* 1998;133:424-8.
- Kips JC, Pauwels RA. Long acting inhaled β2 agonist therapy in asthma. *Am J Respir Crit Care Med* 2001;164:923-32.
- Knorr B, Matz J, Bernstein JA, Nguyen HH, Seidenberg BC, Reiss TF, et al. Montelukast for chronic asthma in 6- to 14-year-old children: a randomized, double-blind trial. *JAMA* 1998;279:1181-6.
- Masoli M, Weatherall M, Holst S, Beasley R. Systematic review of the dose-response relation of inhaled fluticasone propionate. *Arch Dis Child* 2004;89:902-7.
- Patel L, Wales JK, Kibirige MS, Massarano AA, Couriel JM, Clayton PE. Symptomatic adrenal insufficiency during inhaled corticosteroid treatment. *Arch Dis Child* 2001;85:330-4.
- Simons FE, Villa JR, Lee BW, Teper AM, Lyttle B, Aristizabal G, et al. Montelukast added to budesonide in children with persistent asthma: a randomized, double-blind, crossover study. *J Pediatr* 2001;138:694-8.
- Todd GR, Acerini CL, Ross-Russell R, Zahra S, Warner JT, McCance D. Survey of adrenal crisis associated with inhaled corticosteroids in the United Kingdom. *Arch Dis Child* 2002;87:457-61.

15 Acute severe asthma

Parents and children need clear instructions about what to do when an acute asthma attack occurs and when to ask for medical help. If the attack does not respond quickly to the child's usual relief medication (usually two to four puffs of a bronchodilator every 20-30 minutes), treatment should be initiated at home with a large dose of a β_2 agonist bronchodilator. Up to 10 puffs salbutamol or terbutaline by MDI plus spacer, with or without a facemask, with one puff given every 15-30 seconds, or nebulised bronchodilator therapy every 20-30 minutes is advised as a trial of therapy while the family are seeking medical attention.

The response to treatment should be documented objectively in all children old enough to use a peak flow meter. A child who responds well to a high dose of bronchodilator at home will need to be reviewed a few hours later and may require increased prophylactic treatment—either an increase in inhaled steroid therapy or add-on therapy as discussed above. Consideration should be given to starting a course of oral prednisolone at 1-2 mg/kg/day. If the child fails to respond or relapses despite the above management, oral prednisolone, should be started, oxygen should be given, and arrangements made for transfer to hospital.

Indicators of acute severe asthma in children

Child aged <5 years
- Child is too breathless to talk or feed
- Respiratory rate >50 breaths per minute
- Pulse rate >140 beats per minute
- Use of accessory muscles by child

Child aged ≥5 years
- Child is too breathless to talk or feed
- Respiratory >40 breaths per minute
- Pulse rate >120 beats per minute
- Use of accessory muscles by child
- Peak flow <50% best or predicted

Treatment in hospital

The principles of assessment and treatment in hospital of children aged >2 are similar to those for adults, but either local or national guidelines and protocols should be followed. When faced with an intravenous infusion young children sometimes become extremely distressed, which can make their asthma worse. In such cases it may be better to treat them with nebulised salbutamol, ipratropium bromide, and a course of oral steroids.

Oxygen and dehydration

Oxygen is important in treatment but sometimes difficult to give to toddlers. They become dehydrated because of poor fluid intake, sweating, and, in the early stages, hyperventilation. This must be corrected, but there are potential risks of overhydrating children with severe asthma. Production of antidiuretic hormone may be increased during the attack, and the considerable negative intrathoracic pressures generated by the respiratory efforts may predispose to pulmonary oedema. After correcting dehydration the wisest course is to give normal fluid requirements and measure the plasma and urine osmolality.

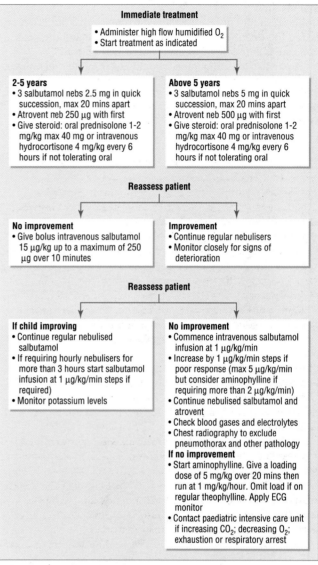

Management of severe asthma in children

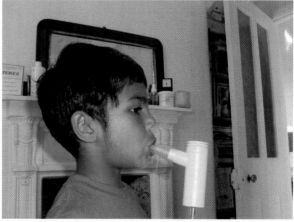

Nebulised therapy being given via mouthpiece during treatment for an acute episode of asthma

Antibiotics

As most asthma attacks in childhood are triggered by viruses and discoloured sputum is often due to inflammatory cells such as eosinophils and neutrophils, there is no role for antibiotics in the management of acute asthma.

Stabilisation

Children should not be discharged from hospital until they are taking the treatment that will be used at home and the peak flow rate is at least 75% of expected or best known.

A paediatric asthma nurse should assess inhaler technique, give general advice and a written asthma action plan, and arrange appropriate follow-up. This can improve the outcome and reduce frequency of readmission to hospital.

Features of life threatening asthma

- Cyanosis, silent chest, poor respiratory effort
- Fatigue or exhaustion
- Agitation or reduced level of consciousness
- Difficulty in speaking
- Peak flow rate <33% best or predicted (in children aged >5)
- Oxygen saturation <92% in room air

Appendix—Personal asthma action plan (with permission from Asthma UK). This plan is intended for use by people aged 12 and above

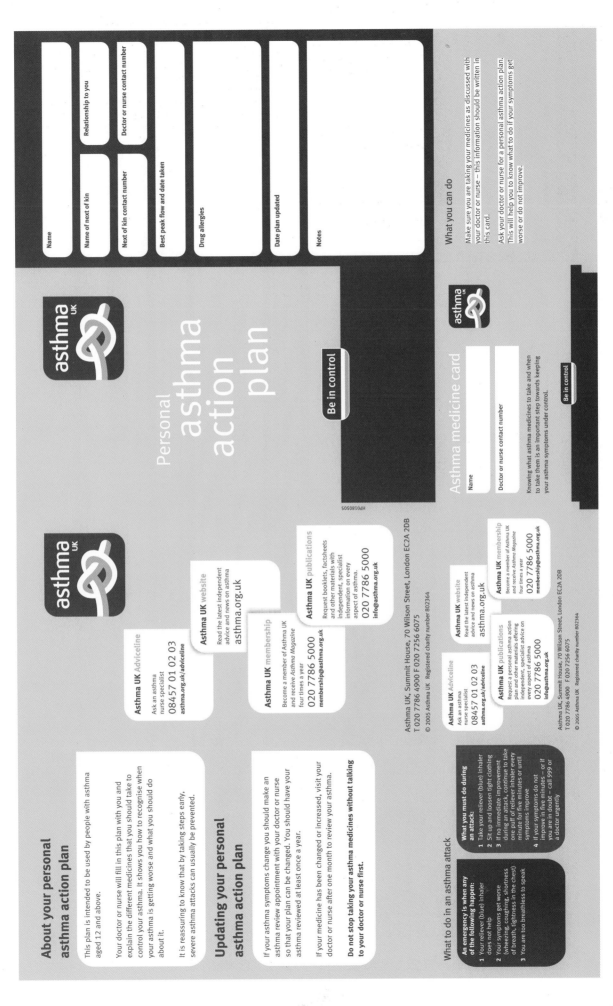

About your personal asthma action plan

This plan is intended to be used by people with asthma aged 12 and above.

Your doctor or nurse will fill in this plan with you and explain the different medicines that you should take to control your asthma. It shows you how to recognise when your asthma is getting worse and what you should do about it.

It is reassuring to know that by taking steps early, severe asthma attacks can usually be prevented.

Updating your personal asthma action plan

If your asthma symptoms change you should make an asthma review appointment with your doctor or nurse so that your plan can be changed. You should have your asthma reviewed at least once a year.

If your medicine has been changed or increased, visit your doctor or nurse after one month to review your asthma.

Do not stop taking your asthma medicines without talking to your doctor or nurse first.

What to do in an asthma attack

An emergency is when any of the following happen:
1 Your reliever (blue) inhaler does not help
2 Your symptoms get worse (wheezing, coughing, shortness of breath, tightness in the chest)
3 You are too breathless to speak

What you must do during an attack:
1 Take your reliever (blue) inhaler
2 Sit up and loosen tight clothing
3 If no immediate improvement during an attack, continue to take one puff of reliever inhaler every minute for five minutes or until symptoms improve
4 If your symptoms do not improve in five minutes— or if you are in doubt— call 999 or a doctor urgently

Asthma UK Adviceline
Ask an asthma nurse specialist
08457 01 02 03
asthma.org.uk/adviceline

Asthma UK website
Read the latest independent advice and news on asthma
asthma.org.uk

Asthma UK membership
Become a member of Asthma UK and receive *Asthma Magazine* four times a year
020 7786 5000
membership@asthma.org.uk

Asthma UK publications
Request booklets, factsheets and other materials with independent, specialist information on every aspect of asthma.
020 7786 5000
info@asthma.org.uk

Asthma UK, Summit House, 70 Wilson Street, London EC2A 2DB
T 020 7786 4900 F 020 7256 6075
© 2005 Asthma UK Registered charity number 802364

Personal asthma action plan

Be in control

Name	
Name of next of kin	**Relationship to you**
Next of kin contact number	**Doctor or nurse contact number**
Best peak flow and date taken	
Drug allergies	
Date plan updated	
Notes	

HP0180505

Asthma medicine card

Be in control

Name

Doctor or nurse contact number

Knowing what asthma medicines to take and when to take them is an important step towards keeping your asthma symptoms under control.

What you can do

Make sure you are taking your medicines as discussed with your doctor or nurse – this information should be written in this card.

Ask your doctor or nurse for a personal asthma action plan. This will help you to know what to do if your symptoms get worse or do not improve.

Asthma UK Adviceline
Ask an asthma nurse specialist
08457 01 02 03
asthma.org.uk/adviceline

Asthma UK publications
Request a personal asthma action plan and other materials offering independent, specialist advice on every aspect of asthma
020 7786 5000
info@asthma.org.uk

Asthma UK website
Read the latest independent advice and news on asthma
asthma.org.uk

Asthma UK membership
Become a member of Asthma UK and receive *Asthma Magazine* four times a year
020 7786 5000
membership@asthma.org.uk

Asthma UK, Summit House, 70 Wilson Street, London EC2A 2DB
T 020 7786 4900 F 020 7256 6075
© 2005 Asthma UK Registered charity number 802364

Zone 1

Your asthma is under control if:

- You have no or minimal symptoms during the day or night (wheezing, coughing, shortness of breath, tightness in the chest)
- You can do all of your normal activities without asthma symptoms
- Your peak flow reading is above [ ] (85% of your best)

Action

Continue to take your usual asthma medicines.

Preventer medicine should be used every day, even when you are feeling well. Your preventer medicine is

name [ ]

colour [ ]   Take [ ] number of puffs/doses

dosage [ ]   when [ ]

Reliever medicine should be used if you have symptoms. Your reliever medicine is

name [ ]

colour [ ]   Take [ ] number of puffs/doses

when [ ]

Other medicines taken regularly may be added to your treatment if your preventer is not stopping all of your symptoms. Your add-on medicine is name [ ]

colour [ ]   Take [ ] number of puffs/doses

when [ ]

If you are always in zone 1, your doctor or nurse may want to reduce (step down) your regular medicines.

Zone 2

Your asthma gets worse if:

- You need to use your reliever inhaler more than once a day
- You have had difficulty sleeping because of your asthma
- Your peak flow reading is between [ ] and [ ] (between 70% and 85% of your best)

Action

Increase your preventer inhaler

name [ ]

colour [ ]   Take [ ] number of puffs/doses

dosage [ ]   when [ ]

Stay on this dose until you have had no symptoms for [ ] days then return to your dose in zone 1.

Continue to take your reliever medicine

name [ ]

colour [ ]   [ ] when needed.

If your symptoms do not improve in [ ] days contact your doctor or nurse for advice.

Your doctor or nurse will discuss your inhaler with you and check your inhaler technique. You may be started on a different medicine to help you get your symptoms back under control.

If you are often in zone 2, let your doctor or nurse know at your next review. Your usual medicines may need to be increased or changed.

Zone 3

Your asthma is much more severe if:

- You need to take your reliever inhaler every four hours or more often
- You have symptoms all the time
- Your peak flow reading is between [ ] and [ ] (between 50% and 70% of your best)

Action

Continue taking your preventer medicine as prescribed at the higher dose in zone 2.

Continue to take your reliever medicine when needed.

If you have been prescribed steroid tablets, take [ ] number 5mg prednisolone tablets immediately and again every morning for [ ] days or until your symptoms have improved or your peak flow has been at [ ] for two days.

Your doctor or nurse may want you to let them know within 24–36 hours that you have started a course of steroid tablets. If you regularly take steroid tablets, your doctor or nurse will advise you on how to reduce the number you are taking.

If you are often in zone 3, let your doctor or nurse know. Your usual medicines may need to be increased or changed.

Zone 4

It is an asthma emergency if any of the following happen:

1 Your reliever (blue) inhaler does not help
2 Your symptoms get worse (cough, breathless, wheeze, tight chest)
3 You are too breathless to speak
4 Your peak flow reading is below [ ]

Action

1 Take your reliever (blue) inhaler

2 Sit up and loosen tight clothing

3 If no immediate improvement during an attack, continue to take one puff/dose of reliever inhaler every minute for five minutes or until symptoms improve

4 If your symptoms do not improve in five minutes – or if you are in doubt – call 999 or a doctor urgently

How to recognise if your asthma is getting worse

Have you had difficulty sleeping because of your asthma symptoms (including coughing)?

Have you had your usual asthma symptoms during the day (wheezing, coughing, shortness of breath, tightness in the chest)?

Has your asthma interfered with your usual activities (eg housework, work or school)?

If **'yes'** to one or more of the above, or if you have not seen your doctor or nurse about your asthma for 12 months or more, arrange to have a review. If **'yes'** to all of the above – is this an emergency? (see overleaf)

Your asthma medicines – what to use on an everyday basis

	Your medicine is:	How much to use:	When to use:	Comments/symptoms:
Preventer				
Reliever				
Other				

Index

Index

Index

Index

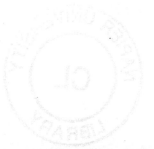